RADIOLOG TECHNIQUES

To Joseph Coral for his achievements

MULTIPLE CHOICE TUTOR

RADIOLOGICAL ANATOMY, PHYSICS AND TECHNIQUES

Anthony Coral MB, MRCP
Registrar in Diagnostic Radiology, St Mary's Hospital, London

and

Allan T. Irvine MB, DMRD, MRCP
Senior Registrar in Diagnostic Radiology, St Mary's Hospital, London

WILLIAM HEINEMANN MEDICAL BOOKS
London

First published 1985
by William Heinemann Medical Books,
23 Bedford Square,
London WC1B 3HH

ISBN: 0–433–06460–9

Photoset by Wilmaset, Birkenhead, Wirral
Printed and bound in Great Britain by
Redwood Burn Ltd., Trowbridge, Wilts.

CONTENTS

FOREWORD

Multiple choice questions are now commonly used in medical examinations. Often candidates find this format difficult; some because of their searching nature, and others because of unfamiliarity with the wide variety of questions and the ways to answer them. This book sets out to help those candidates and, indeed, to widen the knowledge of those who read it. An essential part of this book is the inclusion of reasoned answers with references and this must prove most useful. The authors have experience in multiple choice questions, gained in studying and obtaining their MRCP examinations; and also in studying for the Part I of the FRCR. This book is aimed at Radiologists studying the radiological basic sciences and also at Radiographers needing to study anatomy, radiological physics, radiography and radiological technique.

It is my opinion that this book is a most useful addition to the list of books one should read for the study of these subjects. I can certainly recommend it, and record my great pleasure in being able to write this foreword.

Oscar Craig, FRCSI, FRCS, FRCR
Director
Department of Diagnostic Radiology,
St. Mary's Hospital, London.

PREFACE

Multiple choice questions (MCQs) have an increasing role to play in current medical examinations. This is particularly true in diagnostic radiology and imaging. They provide the examiner with a rapid and objective means of assessing the candidate.

In this book, we have produced nearly 300 five-part questions aimed at the radiologist in training and the radiographer working for higher examinations. Each part of any question may be either true or false. They have been divided conventionally into:

I. Radiological anatomy
II. Radiological physics
III. Radiological techniques and radiography

The questions are of varying difficulty; many are included because they illustrate an important point. Virtually all of the answers are accompanied by an explanation and a reference. These are provided so that the reader can verify the answers and, hopefully, learn from his errors. The major references (*A–Z*) are standard text books in this field. They are listed at the end of the book. References to relevant papers are also included and are cited in full in the answer in which they appear.

We wish to thank the Staff of the Radiology Department at St Mary's Hospital for their help during the writing of the questions. In particular, we wish to thank Dr Graham Cherryman of Aberdeen Royal Infirmary, and Dr Christopher Barber from our own department, for their advice.

London, 1985

AC
ATI

ABBREVIATIONS

The following abbreviations appear in the questions:

CT	= Computed tomography
NMR	= Nuclear magnetic resonance
LMP	= Last menstrual period
IUCD	= Intrauterine contraceptive device
AP	= Anteroposterior
PA	= Posteroanterior
RAO	= Right anterior oblique (i.e. right anterior surface nearer film)
RPO	= Right posterior oblique (i.e. right posterior surface nearer film)
LAO	= Left anterior oblique
LPO	= Left posterior oblique
C1–7	= Cervical vertebra (e.g. C6 is the sixth cervical vertebra)
T or D1–12	= Thoracic vertebra
L1–5	= Lumbar vertebra

I. RADIOLOGICAL ANATOMY

RADIOLOGICAL ANATOMY

1 The diaphragm:

A. Is related anteriorly to the right adrenal.
B. Is attached to the lower six costal cartilages.
C. May normally have a scalloped appearance on a frontal chest radiograph.
D. Has a larger crus on the left than on the right.
E. Has the oesophageal opening in the central tendon.

2 The diaphragm:

A. Has its central tendon more anteriorly placed than posteriorly.
B. May lie at a higher level on the left in a normal chest radiograph.
C. Is pierced by the oesophagus at the level of T8.
D. Is attached to the medial arcuate ligament.
E. Transmits the thoracic duct between the crura.

Answers overleaf

1A
TRUE—Reference *G*, p. 57.

1B
TRUE—Reference *G*, p. 56.

1C
TRUE—This is believed to be caused by irregular contractions of the diaphragmatic musculature. Reference H, p. 640.

1D
FALSE—The left is attached to the upper two lumbar vertebrae and the right to the upper three. Reference *G*, p. 56.

1E
FALSE—It passes through an opening in the muscle of the right crus. Reference *G*, p. 56.

2A
TRUE—It is not, therefore, truly central. Reference *H*, p. 639.

2B
TRUE—Reference *W*, p. 421.

2C
FALSE—This occurs at the level of T10. Reference *G*, p. 56.

2D
TRUE—The ligament passes over psoas from the body of the first lumbar vertebra to its transverse process. Reference *G*, p. 56.

2E
TRUE—Along with the aorta and the azygos vein. Reference *G*, p. 56.

3 Concerning accessory lobes and fissures in the lung:

A. The inferior accessory fissure is the commonest accessory fissure.
B. The inferior accessory fissure occurs more frequently on the left.
C. The posterior basal segment may exist as a separate lobe.
D. A middle lobe on the left occurs in about 2% of normal chests.
E. The superior accessory fissure divides off the apical segment of the lower lobe from the remainder of the lobe.

4 The thoracic duct:

A. Is closely related to the oesophagus.
B. Lies to the right of the azygos vein.
C. Crosses in front of the carotid sheath.
D. Crosses to the left of the median plane at the level of T5.
E. Has no valves.

Answers overleaf

3A
TRUE—This separates the medial basal segment of the lower lobe. It is seen in approximately 8% of frontal chest films and 45% of post-mortem specimens. Reference *H*, p. 611.

3B
FALSE—It occurs more often on the right. Reference *W*, p. 78.

3C
FALSE

3D
FALSE—It practically never occurs. Reference *H*, p. 611.

3E
TRUE—It occurs less frequently than the inferior accessory fissure and more commonly than the azygos fissure. It may be easily mistaken for the minor septum. Reference *W*, p. 77.

4A
TRUE—It is a posterior relation of the oesophagus. Reference *H*, p. 672.

4B
FALSE—It lies to the left of the vein. Reference *G*, p. 92.

4C
FALSE—It crosses behind the sheath. Reference *H*, p. 672.

4D
TRUE—Reference *H*, p. 672.

4E
FALSE—Valves can usually be visualized in the thoracic duct at lymphangiography. They are highly variable in size and number. Reference *H*, p. 689.

5 At the level of the third thoracic vertebra in the chest, the trachea is immediately related to:

A. The thymus.
B. The right phrenic nerve.
C. The right pleura.
D. The brachiocephalic artery.
E. The superior vena cava.

6 In the chest:

A. The left main bronchus is narrower than the right main bronchus.
B. The carinal angle is normally about 60 degrees in adults.
C. There are usually three segments in the left upper lobe.
D. The right pulmonary artery lies above the right main bronchus.
E. The right main bronchus may normally indent the oesophagus.

Answers overleaf

5A
FALSE—The remains of the thymus in the adult are situated in the anterior mediastinum away from the trachea. Reference *H*, p. 663 (Fig. 11-6).

5B
FALSE—This lies lateral to the superior vena cava. Reference *H*, p. 663 (Fig. 11-6).

5C
TRUE—Reference *H*, p. 663 (Fig. 11-6).

5D
TRUE—Reference *H*, p. 663 (Fig. 11-6).

5E
TRUE—The superior vena cava is formed at this level by the union of the brachiocephalic veins. Reference *H*, p. 663 (Fig. 11-6).

6A
TRUE—Because the right main bronchus is wider and more vertically orientated than the left, foreign bodies tend to enter it more frequently. Reference *G*, p. 79.

6B
TRUE—The angle is normally greater in children and gradually diminishes with growth. An enlarged left atrium increases the angle. Reference *H*, p. 594.

6C
FALSE—The usual arrangement (75% of cases) is a bifurcation into a superior division, supplying the apicoposterior and anterior segments; and a lingular division, supplying a superior and an inferior segment. Reference *W*, p. 156.

6D
FALSE—The artery lies anterior to the bronchus. It is the left pulmonary artery that arches over the left main bronchus. Reference *H*, p. 624 (Fig. 10-40).

6E
FALSE—The left main bronchus is one of four points of narrowness in the oesophagus, the others being at the level of the cricoid, at the level of aortic knob and during passage through the diaphragm. Reference *H*, p. 771.

7 In the right lung:

A. The upper lobe usually has four segmental divisions.
B. The apical segmental bronchus of the upper lobe may arise directly from the trachea.
C. A subsuperior segment in the lower lobe is present in 50% of individuals.
D. The minor fissure is seen in 80% of frontal radiographs.
E. The azygos lobe is seen in 5% of frontal radiographs.

8 In the chest:

A. The right oblique fissure is more vertically orientated than the left.
B. The interlobar septa consist of visceral and parietal pleura.
C. The pores of Kohn permit transfer of air between the lobes.
D. The anterior basal branch of the right lower lobe bronchus is usually given off before the medial basal branch.
E. Of an infant, the trachea may normally deviate to the right.

Answers overleaf

7A
FALSE—It usually has three: apical, posterior and anterior. In about 15% of individuals will be found the so-called axillary segment. Reference *W*, p. 151.

7B
TRUE—It is known as a 'displaced bronchus', i.e. a bronchus in an abnormal position which supplies a normally located pulmonary segment. Reference *W*, p. 151.

7C
TRUE—And it is present in about 30% of individuals on the left. Reference *W*, pp. 155-7.

7D
FALSE—Although present in 80% of dissections, it is seen in about 50% of frontal films. Reference *W*, p. 73.

7E
FALSE—It is seen in 1% of anatomic dissections and 0.4% of frontal chest films. Reference *W*, p. 74.

8A
FALSE—The left tends to be the more vertically orientated and to join the diaphragmatic pleura more posteriorly. The approximate angles to the horizontal are 60 degrees for the left and 50 degrees for the right. Reference *H*, p. 609.

8B
FALSE—They consist of two layers of visceral pleura. Reference *H*, p. 638.

8C
FALSE—The pores are openings in the alveoli which permit collateral air drift between segments of the lung only. The canals of Lambert are broncho-alveolar connections. Reference *H*, p. 608.

8D
FALSE—The medial basal branch is given off first at the level of the apical segmental bronchus. Reference *W*, p. 144 (Fig. 4-1).

8E
TRUE—This is thought to be due either to thymic enlargement or to tracheal redundancy. Reference *H*, p. 593.

9 The azygos vein:

A. Is usually formed anterior to the transverse process of L3.
B. Lies immediately anterior to the oesophagus at the level of D8.
C. Receives the oesophageal veins.
D. Receives the inferior thyroid vein.
E. Receives the right lymph trunk.

10 The azygos 'knob' (i.e. that part of the azygos vein that is seen on the frontal view of the chest:)

A. Lies between the right upper lobe and intermediate bronchi.
B. Is enlarged if greater than 10 mm in diameter on an erect film.
C. Is normally larger in pregnancy.
D. Is larger in the erect than in the supine position.
E. Is smaller on inspiration.

Answers overleaf

9A
FALSE—This is too low. The azygos and hemiazygos veins are formed at the level of the renal veins, which is L2. Reference *G*, p. 75.

9B
FALSE—It lies posteriorly and to the right of the oesophagus at this level. Reference *H*, p. 770 (Fig. 13-7).

9C
TRUE—These veins may enlarge in chronic superior vena cava obstruction. Reference *W*, p. 236.

9D
FALSE—This vein unites with its fellow prior to joining the left brachiocephalic vein. Reference *G*, p. 362.

9E
FALSE—This structure drains into the right brachiocephalic vein. Reference *G*, p. 92.

10A
FALSE—It lies between the origin of the right upper lobe bronchus and the right tracheal border. Reference *W*, p. 232.

10B
TRUE—According to Felson, who looked at a large series of normal chest films. Reference *W*, p. 236.

10C
TRUE—Reference *H*, p. 669.

10D
FALSE—It is larger in the supine position. Reference *H*, p. 669.

10E
TRUE—Reference *W*, p. 236.
The fact that the azygos shrinks on standing, on inspiration and during the valsalva manoeuvre permits its differentiation from an enlarged azygos node. Reference *W*, p. 258.

11 The bronchial arteries:

A. Usually arise from the aorta.
B. May arise from the internal mammary arteries.
C. Usually arise at the level of D7–8.
D. Do not normally communicate with the pulmonary circulation.
E. May be seen on a normal chest radiograph.

12 Concerning the normal right descending pulmonary artery:

A. The maximum normal width in men is 20 mm.
B. Width measurements are greater in expiration.
C. Forms an angle with the inferior pulmonary vein which is known as the hilar angle.
D. The hilar angle normally measures 160 degrees.
E. The hilar angle changes with rise in left atrial pressure.

Answers overleaf

11A
TRUE—In 90% of cases. Reference *H*, p. 615.

11B
TRUE—They may also arise from the subclavian or first three intercostal arteries. Reference *H*, p. 615.

11C
FALSE—In 80% of cases they arise at the level of D5–6. Reference *H*, p. 615.

11D
FALSE—The bronchial arteries form capillary plexuses which drain via both bronchial and pulmonary veins. Reference *H*, p. 615.

11E
FALSE—They become enlarged and may be visualized in conditions such as Fallot's tetralogy where pulmonary arterial flow is reduced. Reference *W*, p. 230.

12A
FALSE—According to Chang, the maximum normal width in men is 16 mm and in women 15 mm. Above these measurements, the pulmonary artery is abnormal and pulmonary hypertension should be considered. Reference: The normal roentgenographic measurement of the right descending pulmonary artery in 1085 cases. *Am. J. Roent*; **87**:929–35 (1962).

12B
FALSE—It usually measures 1–2 mm more in inspiration. This is thought to occur because of the fall in intra-alveolar pressure. It may measure more in expiration when pulmonary hypertension is present. Reference: *Am. J. Roent*; **87**:929–35 (1962).

12C
FALSE—The hilar angle is that between the descending pulmonary artery and the superior pulmonary vein. Reference *H*, p. 615.

12D
FALSE—It usually measures 120 degrees. Reference *H*, p. 615.

12E
TRUE—It tends to become obliterated in this situation. Reference *H*, p. 615.

13 The oesophagus:

A. Begins at the level of the fourth cervical vertebra.
B. Is related to the left common carotid artery.
C. Is related to the left recurrent laryngeal nerve.
D. Is related to the right pulmonary artery.
E. Is related to the external jugular vein.

14 Concerning the oesophagus:

A. An aberrant right subclavian artery produces an anterior impression on the oesophagus.
B. It is directly related to the arch of the aorta.
C. Cricopharyngeus may produce an anterior impression in its upper part.
D. Schatzki's ring marks the junction between gastric and oesophageal mucosa.
E. The right atrium is an immediate anterior relation.

Answers overleaf

13A
FALSE—It begins behind the cricoid cartilage at the level of C6. Reference *G*, p. 364.

13B
TRUE—It is related in the neck to the lateral lobes of the thyroid and the common carotid arteries. Reference *G*, p. 364.

13C
TRUE—The nerves lie between the trachea and the oesophagus. Reference *G*, p. 364.

13D
FALSE—It is separated from the artery by the right main bronchus. Reference *H*, p. 770 (Fig. 13-7).

13E
FALSE—The vein lies anteriorly in the neck and is not related. Reference *G*, p. 372.

14A
FALSE—This anomaly which is associated with persistence of a right aortic arch produces a posterior impression on the oesophagus. Reference *H*, p. 697.

14B
TRUE—As the aorta arches backwards towards the vertebral column, it passes to the left side of the oesophagus and causes it to be deviated to the right. Reference *H*, p. 768.

14C
FALSE—The cricopharyngeus produces its impression posteriorly. Reference *H*, p. 784 (Fig. 13-24).

14D
TRUE—Also known as a Wolf B ring, it represents the true mucosal junction when a portion of the stomach has herniated through the diaphragmatic hiatus. Reference *H*, pp. 773–8.

14E
FALSE—In the lower thorax, it is separated from the left atrium by pericardium. Reference *G*, p. 77.

15 The anterior descending branch of the left coronary artery:

A. Is accompanied by the middle cardiac vein.
B. Supplies the interventricular septum.
C. Usually gives a branch to the sino-atrial node.
D. Supplies the anteroapical portion of the left ventricle.
E. Anastomoses with the posterior descending artery over the apex of the heart.

16 In the heart:

A. The right coronary artery arises from the right posterior aortic sinus.
B. The superomedial part of the right atrium is directly related to the root of the aorta.
C. The mitral valve lies anterior to the aortic valve.
D. The tricuspid valve lies posteroinferiorly in the right ventricle.
E. The aortic valve lies posteromedially in relation to the pulmonary valve.

Answers overleaf

15A
FALSE—It is accompanied by the great cardiac vein in the anterior interventricular groove. The middle cardiac vein is situated in the posterior interventricular groove. Reference *H*, p. 750.

15B
TRUE—It supplies the anterior two-thirds of the apical portion of the septum. Reference *H*, p. 746.

15C
FALSE—Although it may do so, it is usual for the node to be supplied from the right coronary artery. Reference *H*, p. 750.

15D
TRUE—Reference *H*, p. 746.

15E
TRUE—And also via septal anastomoses. Reference *H*, p. 758 (Fig. 12-58).

16A
FALSE—It arises from the anterior sinus. The left coronary arises from the left posterior sinus. Reference *G*, p. 62.

16B
TRUE—This is the right auricular appendage. Reference *G*, p. 60.

16C
FALSE—It lies posteriorly and inferiorly. Reference *H*, p. 702 (Fig. 12-13); and p. 698 (Fig. 12-11).

16D
TRUE—Reference *G*, p. 61.

16E
TRUE—Reference *H*, p. 702 (Fig. 12-13); and p. 698 (Fig. 12-11).

17 Veins opening directly into the right atrium include:

A. The coronary sinus.
B. The great cardiac vein.
C. The anterior cardiac veins.
D. The oblique vein.
E. The small cardiac vein.

18 The superior vena cava:

A. Is formed at the middle of the right manubrial border.
B. Enters the right atrium at the level of the fourth costal cartilage.
C. Is directly related to the pleura covering the mediastinal surface of the right lung.
D. Is partly covered by pericardium.
E. Receives the bronchial veins.

Answers overleaf

17A
TRUE—This is formed at the left border of the heart and enters the right atrium near to the orifice of the inferior vena cava. Reference *G*, p. 65.

17B
FALSE—It joins the left marginal vein to form the coronary sinus. Reference *G*, p. 65.

17C
TRUE—These several veins drain the anterior wall of the right ventricle directly into the atrium. Reference *G*, p. 65.

17D
FALSE—It drains into the coronary sinus. Reference *G*, p. 65.

17E
FALSE—It drains into the sinus. Reference *G*, p. 65.

18A
TRUE—Reference *G*, pp. 74–5.

18B
FALSE—It does so at the level of the third costal cartilage. Reference *G*, pp. 74–5.

18C
TRUE—Reference *G*, pp. 74–5.

18D
TRUE—In its lower half it is covered by serous and fibrous pericardium. Reference *G*, pp. 74–5.

18E
FALSE—The superior vena cava receives a single tributary, the azygos vein. The bronchial veins drain into the azygos system. Reference *G*, pp. 74–5.

19 Concerning the paraspinal lines:

A. The right paraspinal line is seen more frequently than the left.
B. The right line usually extends above T6.
C. They are associated with wider paraspinal soft tissues in the elderly.
D. The left paraspinal soft tissues tend to be wider than those on the right.
E. They represent the interface of mediastinal soft tissues and contiguous lung.

20 The aorta:

A. Enters the abdomen at the level of the lower end of T12.
B. Normally divides at the level of L5.
C. Is directly related on its right side to the cisterna chyli.
D. Gives off four unpaired branches.
E. Gives off the gonadal arteries opposite the lower end of L1.

Answers overleaf

19A

FALSE—According to Lien and Kolbenstvedt, the right line is seen in one third, and the left in nearly all cases. Reference: The thoracic paraspinal shadow: normal appearances. Reference: *Clinical Radiology*; **33**:31–5 (1982).

19B

FALSE—It is seen at levels below this. Reference: *Clinical Radiology*; **33**:31–5 (1982).

19C

TRUE—This is related in some way to aortic unfolding. Reference: *Clinical Radiology*; **33**:31–5 (1982).

19D

TRUE—There is a considerable normal range at each level. Depending on which level measurement is made, the mean width on the right varies from 4 to 6 mm and on the left from 5 to 10 mm. Reference: *Clinical Radiology*; **33**:31–5 (1982).

19E

TRUE—Reference: *Clinical Radiology*; **33**:31–5 (1982).
Although the lines may represent layers of parietal and visceral pleura, it seems likely that they are due to the Mach effect. This is a form of edge enhancement which is an illusion created by a retinal reflex. It occurs at boundaries marking a sudden change in tissue densities. Reference: Lane E. J., Proto, A. V. and Phillips, T. W. Mach bands and density perception. *Radiology*; **121**:9–17 (1976).

20A

TRUE—It enters the abdomen through the aortic hiatus in the diaphragm between the crura. Reference *H*, p. 958.

20B

FALSE—It generally ends opposite to L4. Reference *H*, p. 958.

20C

TRUE—Reference *G*, p. 146.

20D

TRUE—These are the coeliac artery, the superior and inferior mesenteric arteries and the median sacral artery. The last branch is given off from the posterior aspect of the aorta at the bifurcation. Reference *G*, p. 147.

20E

FALSE—These are given off at the level of L3. Reference *G*, p. 147.

21 The stomach may receive its blood supply from:

A. The common hepatic artery.
B. The splenic artery.
C. The middle colic artery.
→**D.** The superior mesenteric artery.
E. The inferior mesenteric artery.

22 The superior mesenteric artery:

A. Usually arises at the level of L2.
B. Gives off the superior pancreaticoduodenal artery. T
C. Lies to the right of the vein.
D. Crosses the right gonadal vein.
E. May supply the right lobe of the liver.

Answers overleaf

21A
TRUE—Via the right gastric and the gastroduodenal arteries. The former may arise from the left or, uncommonly, the right hepatic arteries. Reference *H*, p. 834.

21B
TRUE—This is the largest branch of the coeliac axis and supplies the stomach via the left gastro-epiploic and the short gastric arteries. Reference *H*, p. 837.

21C
FALSE—This supplies the transverse colon. Reference *G*, p. 123.

21D
TRUE—This artery may give rise to the splenic or right gastroepiploic arteries. Reference *H*, p. 878.

21E
FALSE—It supplies the left colon, the sigmoid and rectum. Reference *H*, p. 881.

22A
FALSE—It usually arises between 1 and 6 mm below the origin of the coeliac trunk, opposite the mid or lower third of the body of the first lumbar vertebra. However, it may arise at lower levels in a minority of cases. Reference *H*, p. 878.

22B
FALSE—It gives the inferior pancreaticoduodenal which forms an arterial arcade along the head of the pancreas by anastomosing with the superior artery, derived from the gastroduodenal. Reference *H*, p. 808 (Fig. 13-51B and C).

22C
FALSE—It lies to the left. Reference *H*, p. 883.

22D
TRUE—The superior mesenteric artery lies within the mesentery of the small bowel and crosses the inferior vena cava, the right ureter and the right gonadal vessels. Reference *G*, p. 123.

22E
TRUE—The right hepatic artery arises from the superior mesenteric in 14% of cases. Reference *H*, p. 878.

23 Concerning arteries to retroperitoneal organs:

A. The adrenal glands may be supplied directly by branches of the aorta.
B. The adrenal glands receive branches from the dorsal pancreatic artery.
C. The adrenal glands are supplied by the inferior phrenic arteries.
D. Multiple renal arteries are seen in less than 2.5% of the population.
E. Renal arteries may normally produce extrinsic filling defects in the calices.

24 The inferior vena cava:

A. Begins anterior to the body of L5.
B. Lies anterior to the right adrenal gland.
C. Pierces the diaphragm at the level of T10.
D. May be seen on a normal lateral chest film.
E. Has no functioning valves.

Answers overleaf

23A
TRUE—These are known as the middle adrenal arteries. They may be single or multiple on each side. They may also be absent. Reference *H*, p. 990.

23B
FALSE

23C
TRUE—In addition to the middle adrenal and inferior phrenic arteries, the adrenal glands are supplied by branches of the renal arteries. Reference *H*, p. 990.

23D
FALSE—These are a common normal variation (occurring in about 25% of the population). Reference *H*, p. 1010.

23E
TRUE—And occasionally, an accessory renal artery arising from a low position may compress the ureter or pelvis. Reference *H*, p. 1022.

24A
TRUE—Reference *H*, p. 960.

24B
TRUE—Reference *G*, p. 148.

24C
FALSE—It pierces the diaphragm at the level of T8. Reference *H*, p. 960.

24D
TRUE—The inferior vena cava may produce confusing appearances on the lateral film. For example, it may mimic atelectasis (Reference *X*, p. 729 (Fig. 9–172)). Identifying it helps to distinguish the right leaf of the diaphragm, which is related to it, from the left, which is not.

24E
TRUE

25 The following are tributaries of the inferior vena cava:

A. The azygos vein.
B. The third and fourth lumbar veins.
C. The right adrenal vein.
D. The left testicular vein.
E. The pancreatic veins.

26 In the normal abdomen, the following structures may be seen on the plain radiograph:

A. The ligamentum teres.
B. The right crus of the diaphragm.
C. The antrum of the stomach simulating a soft-tissue mass.
D. The transversus abdominis muscle.
E. The gall bladder.

Answers overleaf

25A
FALSE—The azygos vein is formed either as a branch of the inferior vena cava or by the union of right ascending lumbar and subcostal veins. It is the tributary of the superior vena cava. Reference *G*, p. 75.

25B
TRUE—The vessels from the left side pass posterior to the aorta. The first and second lumbar veins drain into the ascending lumbar vein, while the fifth drains via the iliolumbar vein into the common iliac. Reference *P*2, p. 197.

25C
TRUE—Reference *G*, p. 148.

25D
FALSE—The left testicular and adrenal veins drain into the left renal vein. The corresponding veins on the right drain into the vena cava. Reference *G*, p. 148.

25E
FALSE—These drain into the splenic vein. Reference *G*, p. 883.

26A
TRUE—Because it may contain fat. By recognizing its characteristic shape and position, it will not be confused with air either in the biliary tree or free in the peritoneum. Reference: Haswell, D. M., Berne, A. S. and Schneider, B. Plain film recognition of the ligamentum teres hepatis. *Radiology*; **114**:263–7 (1975).

26B
TRUE—However, the left is more commonly visible. Reference *X*, p. 771 (Fig. 11-37).

26C
TRUE—Reference *X*, p. 764 (Fig. 11-24).

26D
TRUE—As may the external and internal oblique muscles. This is more often possible in patients with a large amount of body fat. Reference *H*, p. 941 (Fig. 15-19).

26E
FALSE—This is because the visibility of abdominal organs depends on whether they indent the extraperitoneal perivisceral fat or not. The gall bladder does not indent the fat and is therefore not normally visible. It may be detected by its impression on the adjacent transverse colon. Reference: Whalen, J. P. and Berne, A.S. The extraperitoneal perivisceral fat pad. *Radiology*; **92**:466–72 (1969).

27 In the normal abdomen:

A. Unilateral absence of the psoas shadow on a plain film is not seen.
B. The ileocaecal valve may simulate a polypoid mass at barium enema.
C. The spleen does not indent the stomach at a barium meal.
D. Jejunum has an average diameter of 4–4.5 cm.
E. The left lobe of the liver may produce a soft-tissue shadow in the stomach.

28 In the large intestine:

A. The plicae semilunares consist of mucosa only.
B. The absence of haustral pattern in the descending colon signifies a diseased colon.
C. A spiculated appearance in the wall of the sigmoid colon may be due to the normal filling of the mucosal glands of Lieberkühn.
D. The transverse mesocolon is attached to the pancreas.
E. The splenic flexure is highly variable in position.

Answers overleaf

27A

FALSE—Elkin and Cohen found it to be absent on the right in 9%, and on the left in 5.5%, of plain films of normal patients taken prior to intravenous urography. They did not find it to be a reliable indicator of disease. Reference: Diagnostic value of the psoas shadow. *Clinical Radiology*; **13**:210–17 (1962).

27B

TRUE—Reference *X*, p. 811 (Fig. 11-122).
In these cases, it is important to take films demonstrating the relationship to the terminal ileum.

27C

FALSE—Reference *X*, p. 785 (Fig. 11-66). It may mimic a mass.

27D

FALSE—The normal diameter of jejunum is 3–3.5 cm. Ileum is smaller with an average diameter of 2.5 cm or less. Reference *H*, p. 844.

27E

TRUE—Reference *X*, p. 782 (Fig. 11-62). It may mimic a gastric tumour.

28A

FALSE—They consist of submucosa and mucosa. This differs from the valvulae conniventes of the duodenum and jejunum, which consist of mucosa only. Reference *H*, p. 855.

28B

FALSE—Although this is an associated feature of ulcerative colitis, it is not infrequently seen in the normal person. Reference *H*, p. 855.

28C

TRUE—An appearance which is not to be confused with ulcerative colitis. Reference *H*, p. 860.

28D

TRUE—The long mesentery of the transverse colon allows for great variability in its position. However, the first few centimetres are usually firmly attached to the duodenum and pancreatic head, so that enlargement of these structures may cause a secondary displacement of this part of the colon. Reference *H*, p. 849.

28E

FALSE—It tends to hold a constant position because of its attachment to the diaphragm via the phrenicocolic ligament. Reference *H*, p. 849.

29 The rectum:

A. Begins anterior to the lumbosacral articulation.
B. Is related posteriorly to the median sacral artery.
C. Usually has 3–5 crescentic folds known as the valves of Houston.
D. May be separated from the lowermost sacral segment by a presacral width of 2 cm in the normal patient with a barium-filled rectum.
E. Is not related to peritoneum.

Answers overleaf

29A
FALSE—It begins in front of the third sacral segment. Reference *G*, p. 157.

29B
TRUE—It is also related posteriorly to the lateral sacral vessels, the 3rd, 4th and 5th sacral nerves, the sympathetic trunk and the superior rectal artery. Reference *G*, p. 157.

29C
TRUE—Also known as the plicae transversales, these folds are variable in position. They may be poorly developed or absent in an individual patient. Reference *H*, pp. 850–1.

29D
FALSE—When Crispin and Fry measured the presacral space at this level in 100 patients, they found a normal range of 0.2–1.6 cm. Over 1.5 cm was thought suspicious. Over 2 cm was thought definitely abnormal. An undercouch tube was used for exposing the films. The rectum falls away from the sacral concavity when empty, so measurements must be made when distended with barium. Reference: The presacral space shown by barium enema. *British Journal of Radiology*; **36**:319–22 (1963).

29E
FALSE—The upper third is covered by peritoneum on its front and sides. The middle third is related to peritoneum on its front only. The pouch of peritoneum so formed is the rectovesical in the male and the recto-uterine in the female. Reference *G*, p. 157.

30 The portal vein:

A. Is usually formed by the union of inferior mesenteric and splenic veins.
B. Lies posterior to the common hepatic artery.
C. Receives into its left branch the para-umbilical veins.
D. Receives the right gastroepiploic vein.
E. Receives the left gastric (coronary) vein.

31 The common bile duct:

A. Lies posterior to the portal vein.
B. Is closely related to the superior mesenteric artery.
C. Is related to the left hepatic vein.
D. Lies to the right of the gastroduodenal artery.
E. May normally produce a smooth indentation in the barium-filled duodenal cap.

Answers overleaf

30A
FALSE—It begins at the union of superior mesenteric and splenic veins. Reference *G*, p. 125.

30B
TRUE—Anterior to the portal vein in the free edge of the lesser omentum lie the bile duct to the right and the hepatic artery to the left. Reference *G*, p. 125.

30C
TRUE—The para-umbilical veins are a route by which blood can bypass an obstructed intrahepatic portal system. Reference *H*, p. 884.

30D
FALSE—This drains into the superior mesenteric vein before the formation of the portal vein. Reference *H*, p. 883.

30E
TRUE—Reference *G*, p. 125. The communication of the left gastric vein with the oesophageal veins and the azygos system provides a route of bypass of the intrahepatic portal system. Reference *H*, p. 884.

31A
FALSE—The vein lies posterior to the duct in the free edge of the lesser omentum. Reference *G*, p. 133.

31B
FALSE—The duct lies along the left margin of the second part of the duodenum. The artery lies further to the left. Reference *H*, p. 795 (Fig. 13-35B).

31C
FALSE—The hepatic veins are entirely intrahepatic and do not parallel the course of the bile duct within the liver. Reference *H*, p. 883.

31D
TRUE—Reference *G*, p. 133.

31E
TRUE—Reference *X*, p. 799 (Fig. 11-98). The bile duct lies posteriorly so that this effect will occur in the supine position.

32 The pancreas:

A. Originates from a ventral and a dorsal bud.
B. Is retroperitoneal.
C. Lies immediately anterior to the coeliac artery.
D. Normally has a main duct which measures between 5 and 6 mm in diameter.
E. Lies anterior to the portal vein.

33 The head of the pancreas:

A. Has an uncinate process which is crossed by the superior mesenteric artery.
B. Receives its main blood supply from the left gastric artery.
C. Lies directly anterior to the right renal vein.
D. Lies anterior to the inferior vena cava.
E. Has a minor or accessory duct which opens into the duodenum 3 cm distal to the main duct.

Answers overleaf

32A
TRUE—The ventral bud arises in common with the liver. The dorsal bud arises proximal to it. The major duct is derived from both elements, whereas the minor duct derives from the dorsal bud only. Reference *G*, p. 137.

32B
TRUE—Reference *G*, p. 104 (Fig. 9.4A).

32C
FALSE—This is usually at a higher level than the pancreas. Reference *G*, p. 136.

32D
FALSE—This is too wide. The maximum diameter of the duct in the head of the normal gland is 3.9 mm. It narrows as it extends towards the tail. Reference *H*, pp. 830–1.

32E
TRUE—The neck of the gland is related anteriorly. Reference *G*, p. 136.

33A
TRUE—So does the superior mesenteric vein. Reference *H*, p. 823.

33B
FALSE—It is supplied in a variable manner by branches of the splenic, gastroduodenal and pancreaticoduodenal arteries. Reference *H*, p. 825.

33C
TRUE—Reference *G*, p. 136.

33D
TRUE—Reference *H*, p. 823.

33E
FALSE—It opens proximal to the main duct. Reference *G*, p. 136.

34 The right ureter:

A. Passes posterior to the right common iliac artery.
B. Is crossed anteriorly by the right colic and ileocolic arteries.
C. Is related to the lateral aspect of psoas major.
D. Is related to the root of the sigmoid mesocolon.
E. Becomes intraperitoneal in the pelvis.

35 In the normal duodenum:

A. The major papilla opening into the second part may produce a filling defect.
B. The second part is suspended from the diaphragm by the ligament of Treitz.
C. The cap may be indented by the gall bladder.
D. The second part may be displaced medially by the right kidney.
E. The fourth part ascends medial to the inferior mesenteric vein.

Answers overleaf

34A
FALSE—It passes anterior to the artery. Reference *H*, p. 1011.

34B
TRUE—Reference *H*, p. 1011.

34C
FALSE—It is embedded on the medial aspect of the muscle. Reference *H*, p. 1011. Hypertrophy of the muscle in young males may displace the normal ureter medially and mimic retroperitoneal fibrosis. Reference *X*, p. 878 (Fig. 13-48); and p. 879 (Fig. 13-50).

34D
FALSE—This applies to the left ureter. Reference *G*, p. 141.

34E
FALSE—It is an extraperitoneal structure.

35A
TRUE—It may be confused with a tumour. Reference *H*, p. 803 (Fig. 13-46).

35B
FALSE—This attaches the duodenojejunal flexure to the right crus of the diaphragm. Reference *H*, p. 794.

35C
TRUE—Reference *H*, p. 792. This tends to occur in the prone position.

35D
TRUE—Reference *X*, p. 801 (Fig. 11-101).

35E
TRUE—Reference *G*, p. 115.

36 The horizontal (third) part of the duodenum:

A. Lies anterior to the superior mesenteric vessels.
B. Lies anterior to the right ureter.
C. Lies anterior to the inferior vena cava and aorta.
D. Is an intraperitoneal structure.
E. Has no circular mucosal folds (valvulae conniventes).

37 Concerning the peritoneal reflections and spaces:

A. The right subhepatic space communicates directly with the right subphrenic space.
B. There is no communication between the right paracolic gutter and the right subhepatic space.
C. The lesser sac communicates directly with the left infracolic space via the epiploic foramen.
→**D.** The lesser sac is related posteriorly to the left kidney.
E. The lesser sac is related posteriorly to the right adrenal.

Answers overleaf

36A
FALSE—It lies posteriorly to the vessels; the pancreas lies anteriorly. This helps in identifying the pancreas at CT. Reference *G*, p. 115.

36B
TRUE—Reference *G*, p. 115.

36C
TRUE—The gonadal arteries also lie posteriorly. Reference *G*, p. 115.

36D
FALSE—It is retroperitoneal. It is crossed by the root of the small bowel mesentery. Reference *H*, p. 794.

36E
FALSE—These begin in the second part of the duodenum and gradually become more prominent. They are distinctly seen from the duodenal papilla onwards. They usually project about 8 mm into the lumen. Reference *H*, p. 794.

37A
TRUE—They communicate over the right lobe of the liver. The former space is also referred to as Morisson's pouch. Reference *H*, p. 948 (Fig. 15-31).

37B
FALSE—Hence an abscess may spread from the right upper abdomen to the pelvis and vice versa. Reference *H*, p. 946.

37C
FALSE—The lesser sac, which may be thought of as part of the left subhepatic space, passes into the area of Morisson's pouch through the epiploic foramen. The left infracolic space results from the division of the inferior mesocolic space by the root of the mesentery of small bowel. Reference *H*, p. 948.

37D
TRUE—Reference *H*, p. 932.

37E
FALSE—It is related to the left adrenal. It is also related posteriorly to the pancreas and diaphragm. Reference *H*, p. 932.

38 In the liver:

A. The ligamentum teres is the remnant of the umbilical artery.
B. The falciform ligament separates the right and left subhepatic spaces.
C. The caudate lobe is directly related to the first part of the duodenum.
D. The quadrate lobe is separated from the caudate process by the inferior vena cava.
E. The lesser omentum is attached to the interlobar fissure.

39 The epiploic foramen is bounded by:

A. The duodenum.
B. The aorta.
C. The caudate process of the liver.
D. The inferior vena cava.
E. The transverse mesocolon.

40 The spleen:

A. May normally be identified on a plain abdominal film.
B. Is invested in peritoneum.
C. Is related to the tail of the pancreas.
D. Lies on the phrenicocolic ligament.
E. Receives its blood supply via the gastrosplenic ligament.

Answers overleaf

38A
FALSE—It is the remnant of the obliterated umbilical vein. Reference *G*, p. 128.

38B
FALSE—It separates the subphrenic spaces. Reference *G*, p. 129.

38C
FALSE—The quadrate lobe is related to the first part of the duodenum. Reference *G*, p. 131.

38D
FALSE—It is the porta hepatis which intervenes between them. Reference *G*, p. 128 (Fig. 11.1).

38E
TRUE—Reference *G*, p. 129.

39A
TRUE—The first part. Reference *G*, p. 104.

39B
FALSE—Reference *G*, p. 104 (Fig. 9.4B).

39C
TRUE—Reference *G*, p. 131.

39D
TRUE—Reference *G*, p. 104.

39E
FALSE—Reference *G*, p. 104 (Fig. 9.4A).

40A
TRUE—It forms a tongue-like shadow along the left upper lateral aspect of the stomach. Reference *H*, p. 986.

40B
TRUE—Reference *G*, p. 134.

40C
TRUE—This lies in the lienorenal (phrenicosplenic) ligament. Reference *G*, p. 134.

40D
TRUE—This is one of three supporting ligaments. Reference *H*, p. 982.

40E
FALSE—The splenic artery and vein run in the lienorenal ligament to the hilum of the spleen. Reference *H*, p. 982.

41 The anterior relations of the right kidney include:

A. The descending part of the duodenum.
B. The pylorus of the stomach.
C. The liver.
D. The superior mesenteric artery.
E. The hepatic flexure.

42 The left kidney:

A. Usually lies lower than the right.
B. Is usually larger than the right.
C. Is related to the tail of the pancreas.
D. Is related anteriorly to jejunum.
E. Is drained by the main left renal vein which crosses the aorta above the origin of the superior mesenteric artery.

Answers overleaf

41A
TRUE—Reference *G*, p. 138.

41B
FALSE—The left kidney, but not the right, forms part of the stomach bed. Reference *G*, p. 112.

41C
TRUE—The visceral surface of the liver forms the major anterior relation of the right kidney. Reference *G*, p. 138.

41D
FALSE—Reference *G*, p. 123.

41E
TRUE—The lateral aspect of the lower pole is related to colon. Reference *H*, p. 1009 (Fig. 16-13C).

42A
FALSE—The right usually lies lower because of the presence of the liver. Reference *G*, p. 138.

42B
TRUE—However, the difference is normally less than 1 cm. Reference *H*, p. 998.

42C
TRUE—Reference *G*, p. 138.

42D
TRUE—Reference *G*, p. 138.

42E
FALSE—The vein usually passes anterior to the aorta below the level of the superior mesenteric artery. Reference *H*, p. 1006.

43 The urinary bladder:

A. Is supplied by the vesical branches of the external iliac artery.
B. Is attached to the umbilicus by the median umbilical ligament.
C. Is related superiorly to the uterus in the female.
D. Is surrounded by fat.
E. Has a ridge on its internal surface between the ureteric orifices.

44 Concerning the uterus:

A. It is supplied solely by the uterine artery.
B. Lymph drainage is partly to superficial inguinal nodes.
C. It is supported and stabilized by the round ligament.
D. The vaginal fornix lies between the cervix lying medially and the ureters lying laterally.
E. Peritoneum is reflected from it to form the round ligament.

Answers overleaf

43A

FALSE—The superior and inferior vesical arteries are branches of the internal iliac. Reference *G*, p. 161.

43B

TRUE—The ligament is attached to the bladder apex. Reference *G*, p. 160.

43C

TRUE—Reference *G*, p. 161. The uterus commonly makes an impression on the contrast-filled bladder in the normal patient.

43D

TRUE—Reference *H*, p. 1012. This may permit the visualization of the bladder on a plain film and of the bladder wall when the bladder is contrast filled.

43E

TRUE—The interureteric ridge marks the base of the triangular area of smooth mucous membrane known as the trigone. Reference *H*, p. 1014.

44A

FALSE—The uterine artery arises from the internal iliac and anastomoses with the ovarian artery, which arises from the aorta at the level of L3. Reference *G*, p. 163.

44B

TRUE—Via the round ligament. The principal route of drainage is to iliac nodes, however. Reference *G*, p. 163.

44C

FALSE—This is done by the parametrial ligaments (uterosacral, cardinal, and pubocervical). The round ligaments help to maintain anteversion. Reference *G*, p. 163.

44D

TRUE—Reference *G*, p. 163.

44E

FALSE—It forms the broad ligament. The round ligament is derived from the gubernaculum. Reference *G*, p. 162.

45 In the larynx:

→ **A.** The rima glottidis is the area between the vestibular folds.
B. There is a synovial joint between the arytenoid and cricoid cartilages.
C. The vocal ligaments are attached to the thyroid cartilage.
D. The hyaline cartilages tend to calcify.
→ **E.** The ventricle forms a part of the subglottic area.

46 Relating to the larynx:

A. It has a high position in the neonate.
B. The epiglottis produces a central ovoid filling defect in a barium swallow in frontal projection.
C. It is related to the carotid sheath.
→ **D.** The vestibule lies between the false and the true cords.
E. It is developed from foregut.

Answers overleaf

45A
FALSE—It is the elongated slit-like opening between the vocal folds (true vocal cords). It is the narrowest part of the laryngeal cavity. Reference *H*, p. 587.

45B
TRUE—Reference *G*, p. 340.

45C
TRUE—The vocal ligament is the thickened free edge of the conus elasticus. Reference *P*1, p. 173.

45D
TRUE—The thyroid, cricoid and greater part of the arytenoid cartilages are hyaline which tends to calcify. This calcification is frequently irregular, in which case the uncalcified areas should not be misinterpreted as areas of erosion. Also, they should not be confused with foreign bodies. This distinction may be made at barium swallow. Reference *H*, p. 584.

45E
FALSE—The ventricle of the larynx (also known as the sinus) is formed by lateral outpouchings beneath the false cords. It is immediately above the vocal folds, and therefore supraglottic. Reference *H*, p. 587.

46A
TRUE—In a fetus of 6 months, the larynx is situated in a position two vertebrae higher than in an adult. It gradually descends as age increases. Reference *H*, p. 587.

46B
TRUE—Reference *H*, p. 587.

46C
TRUE—The sheath lies laterally. Reference *G*, p. 338.

46D
FALSE—The vestibule lies between the false cords (vestibular folds) inferiorly and the laryngeal aditus superiorly. Reference *H*, p. 586.

46E
TRUE—It arises from the 6th pharyngeal arch on the walls of the primitive foregut. Reference *G*, p. 337.

47 The pyriform fossa:

A. Lies between the tongue and the epiglottis.
B. Is related medially to the arytenoid cartilage.
C. Is bounded partly by the thyrohyoid membrane.
D. Is innervated by the recurrent laryngeal nerve.
E. Communicates with the ventricle of the larynx.

48 The thyroid gland:

A. Derives its blood supply from the internal carotid artery.
B. Has a single large vein draining into the internal jugular vein.
C. Is related to the sternohyoid muscle.
D. Is closely related to the recurrent laryngeal nerve.
E. Is enclosed in pretracheal fascia.

Answers overleaf

47A
FALSE—The valleculae are hollow pockets which lie to each side of the median plane between the dorsum of the tongue and the epiglottis. Reference *H*, p. 582.

47B
TRUE—The fossa lies between the lamina of the thyroid cartilage laterally and the aryepiglottic fold medially. Reference *G*, p. 335.

47C
TRUE—The part of the fossa which lies above the lamina of the thyroid is so bounded. Reference *P*1, p. 169.

47D
FALSE—It is innervated by the internal branch of the superior laryngeal nerve. Reference *P*1, p. 177.

47E
FALSE

48A
FALSE—The internal carotid artery has no branches in the neck. The gland is supplied by the superior and inferior thyroid arteries which are branches of the external carotid and thyrocervical arteries respectively. Reference *G*, p. 362.

48B
FALSE—The venous drainage is via the superior and middle thyroid veins, which are tributaries of the internal jugular, and via the inferior thyroid vein which drains into the left brachiocephalic vein. Reference *G*, p. 362.

48C
TRUE—This is an anterior relation. Reference *G*, p. 362.

48D
TRUE—The nerve lies between the trachea and oesophagus and is a medial relation of the thyroid. Reference *G*, p. 362.

48E
TRUE—Reference *G*, p. 362.

49 In the neck:

A. The posterior atlanto-occipital membrane is the continuation of the posterior longitudinal ligament.
B. The anterior atlanto-occipital membrane is the continuation of the anterior longitudinal ligament.
C. The distance between the anterior margin of the dens and the posterior margin of the anterior arch of the atlas (the atlanto-dental interval) is usually about 1 mm.
D. The atlantodental interval does not change with flexion in the normal patient.
E. The atlanto-axial joints are the joints of Luschka.

50 In the neck:

A. The retropharyngeal space at C2 normally measures 5–8 mm.
B. The spinous process of C7 is usually bifid.
C. The ligamentum nuchae is attached to the spinous processes and occipital bone.
D. A midline anastomosis may occur between the superior thyroid arteries.
E. Scalenus anterior lies anterior to the subclavian vein.

Answers overleaf

49A

FALSE—The posterior atlanto-occipital membrane is the continuation of the ligamentum flavum. The continuation of the posterior longitudinal ligament between the axis and the occipital bone is the membrana tectoria. Reference *P*3, pp. 141–2.

49B

TRUE—The anterior ligament is attached to the vertebral bodies and intervertebral discs. It tapers superiorly to be attached to the anterior tubercle of the atlas, and then continues to the base of the skull anterior to the foramen magnum as the anterior atlanto-occipital membrane. Reference *P*3, p. 141.

49C

TRUE—The mean (±SD) value in adults is 0.93 ± 0.36 mm. Reference *H*, p. 537. The normal range may be considered to be 0.5–3 mm in adults.

49D

FALSE—Flexion tends to increase the interval. Reference *H*, p. 537.

49E

FALSE—The joints of Luschka are synovial joints between the posterolateral margins of the bodies of the lower five cervical vertebrae. Reference *H*, p. 511. They are seen on the PA view of the cervical spine. Reference *H*, p. 540 (Fig. 9-32).

50A

FALSE—It should not normally measure more than 4.5 mm. Reference *H*, p. 588 (Fig. 10-7).

50B

FALSE—However, the spinous processes of C2 to C6 tend to be bifid to some degree. Reference *H*, p. 534.

50C

TRUE—Reference *G*, p. 361. Calcification of the ligament may be seen on a lateral radiograph of the neck, and may be mistaken for a fractured spinous process. Reference *X*, p. 214 (Fig. 3-114).

50D

TRUE—Connecting the external carotid arteries. Reference *H*, p. 360 (Fig. 8-9).

50E

FALSE—It lies posterior to the vein. Reference *G*, p. 361.

51 In the skull of the neonate:

A. Overlapping of the bones of the vault is a sign of serious intracranial damage.
B. Inner and outer tables cannot be differentiated from each other.
C. The spheno-occipital synchondrosis closes at 18 months.
D. A 'J'-shaped pituitary is a normal variation.
E. The metopic suture is best seen in the lateral projection.

52 In the mandible:

A. The symphysis menti is ossified at birth.
B. The mental foramen opens opposite the second incisor.
C. The mylohyoid groove (line) crosses perpendicular to the mandibular canal.
D. The mental spine marks the attachment of geniohyoid.
E. The angle decreases from early adulthood to old age.

Answers overleaf

51A
FALSE—This is seen in a normal situation. Reference *E*, p. 1085.

51B
TRUE—Reference *E*, p. 1086.

51C
FALSE—This ordinarily closes by the 25th year. Reference *H*, p. 255.

51D
TRUE—This refers to a shallow anterior convexity in the sella which is thought to be an exaggeration of the normal slight impression due to the chiasmatic sulcus. Reference *E*, p. 1082.

51E
FALSE—The frontal bone is normally divided at birth by a midline suture, the frontal suture. It is normally obliterated by the fifth or sixth year of life. It is called the metopic suture when it persists into adulthood. (Reference *H*, p. 256). It is seen on the PA view (Reference *H*, p. 253; Fig. 6-35).

52A
FALSE—It ossifies during the second year of life. Reference *G*, p. 301.

52B
FALSE—It opens at the level of the interval between the premolar teeth. (Reference *G*, p. 301). It may be mistaken for an apical abscess (Reference *X*, p. 153; Fig. 2-72).

52C
FALSE—They run a parallel course. The mandibular canal transmits the inferior alveolar nerve and vessels. (Reference *H*, p. 220). The canal is frequently visible on plain films of the mandible.

52D
TRUE—Reference *G*, p. 326.

52E
FALSE—The angle increases in association with the changes in the alveolar margin resulting from the loss of teeth. It changes from about 110 degrees in the adult to about 140 degrees in the elderly. Reference *G*, p. 302.

53 The temporomandibular joint:

A. Is formed between the coronoid process of the mandible and the mandibular fossa.
B. Has a single cavity.
C. Is related to the parotid gland.
D. Is related medially to the sphenomandibular ligament.
→**E.** Is less stable with the mouth open because the condyle lies on the articular tubercle.

54 The following structures lie in the medial wall of the inner ear:

A. The spur or scutum.
B. The chorda tympani.
C. The promontary.
D. The fenestra vestibuli (oval window).
E. The handle of the malleus.

Answers overleaf

53A
FALSE—It is formed with the condyle of the mandible. Reference *G*, p. 331.

53B
FALSE—It is completely divided into superior and inferior compartments by a fibrocartilaginous disc. Each compartment is synovium-lined. Reference *G*, p. 331.

53C
TRUE—Reference *G*, p. 332.

53D
TRUE—This accessory ligament passes from the sphenoid spine to the lingula of the mandible. Reference *G*, p. 332.

53E
TRUE—Reference *G*, p. 332.

54A
FALSE—This refers to a bony projection which forms the superior attachment of the tympanic membrane. Reference *H*, p. 321.

54B
FALSE—It lies between the tympanic membrane and the handle of the malleus laterally and the incus medially. Reference *G*, p. 344.

54C
TRUE—This is the central bulge in the medial wall caused by the first turn of the cochlea. Reference *G*, p. 344.

54D
TRUE—Superiorly and posteriorly to the promontary. It is closed by the footplate of the stapes. Reference *G*, p. 344.

54E
FALSE—Reference *G*, p. 344.

55 In the middle ear:

A. The arcuate eminence forms the roof.
B. The stapedius muscle arises from the promontary.
C. The fenestra vestibuli lies above the fenestra cochleae (round window).
D. The aditus is an opening in the superior part of the posterior wall which communicates with the mastoid antrum.
E. The head of the malleus is attached to the tympanic membrane.

56 The temporal bone:

A. Is entirely situated in the middle cranial fossa.
B. Forms part of the foramen lacerum.
C. Has the falx cerebri attached to it.
D. Transmits the facial nerve.
E. Articulates with the zygomatic bone.

Answers overleaf

55A
FALSE—The thin bony roof of the middle ear is formed by the tegmen tympani. The arcuate eminence lies more medially and encloses the superior semicircular canal. Reference *H*, p. 319.

55B
FALSE—It passes from the pyramid, a bony projection on the posterior wall. Reference *G*, p. 344.

55C
TRUE—Reference *G*, p. 344.

55D
TRUE—Reference *G*, p. 344.

55E
FALSE—The head of the malleus lies in the epitympanic recess; the handle is that part attached to the tympanic membrane. Reference *G*, p. 344.

56A
FALSE—It forms part of the floor of the middle and posterior cranial fossae. Reference *G*, p. 304.

56B
TRUE—The foramen is situated at the junction of the petrous apex, the basilar occipital bone and the sphenoid. Reference *H*, p. 233.

56C
FALSE—The tentorium cerebelli is attached to the superior border of the petrous temporal bone. Reference *G*, p. 423.

56D
TRUE—In the internal auditory canal and in a bony canal within the middle ear. The nerve leaves the bone via the stylomastoid foramen. Reference *G*, p. 354.

56E
TRUE—The zygomatic process of the temporal bone extends forward to contribute to the zygomatic arch. Reference *G*, p. 303.

57 The following structures pass through the parotid gland:

→**A.** The retromandibular vein.
B. The external carotid artery.
→**C.** The internal carotid artery.
D. The lingual nerve.
E. The facial nerve.

58 In the nose:

A. The nasolacrimal duct opens into the inferior meatus.
→**B.** The deep surface of the nasal bones is grooved by the anterior ethmoidal nerves.
C. The maxillary sinus opens into the inferior meatus.
D. The ethmoid air cells lie between the nose and orbit.
E. The frontal sinuses open into the superior meatus.

Answers overleaf

57A
TRUE—Formed behind the neck of the mandible by the joining of superficial temporal and maxillary veins, the retromandibular vein passes through the gland and divides below it into anterior and posterior divisions. Reference *G*, p. 371.

57B
TRUE—The artery lies deep within the gland. Reference *G*, p. 327.

57C
FALSE—It passes medially to the gland. Reference *G*, p. 329 (Fig. 26-9).

57D
FALSE—Reference *G*, p. 353.

57E
TRUE—It divides within the gland. Reference *G*, p. 354.

58A
TRUE—Reference *G*, p. 317.

58B
TRUE—And these may be seen on the lateral view of the nasal bones. Reference *H*, p. 288; and p. 291 (Fig. 7-4).

58C
FALSE—It opens into the middle meatus. Reference *G*, p. 318.

58D
TRUE—Reference *G*, p. 320.

58E
FALSE—The frontal sinuses open into the middle meatus. Reference *G*, p. 318.

59 The ethmoid bone articulates with:

→ **A.** The nasal bone.
B. The palatine bone.
C. The lacrimal bone.
D. The maxilla.
E. The vomer.

60 The ethmoid bone takes part in:

A. The septum of the nose.
B. The hard palate.
C. The attachment of the falx cerebri.
D. The medial wall of the orbit.
E. The lateral wall of the nose.

Answers overleaf

59A
FALSE—The nasal bone articulates superiorly with the frontal bone and laterally with the frontal process of the maxilla. Reference *H*, p. 219 (Fig. 6-5).

59B
TRUE—Reference *H*, p. 219 (Fig. 6-5).

59C
TRUE—Reference *H*, p. 219 (Fig. 6-5).

59D
TRUE—Reference *H*, p. 219.

59E
TRUE—Reference *G*, p. 306.

60A
TRUE—The perpendicular plate of the ethmoid participates with the vomer in forming the bony part of the nasal septum. Reference *H*, p. 289.

60B
FALSE—This is formed by the palatine processes of the maxillae and the horizontal plates of the palatine bones. Reference *H*, p. 236 (Fig. 6-26).

60C
TRUE—The crista galli, which forms the anteroinferior attachment of the falx, is the upward extension of the perpendicular plate of the ethmoid bone. Reference *G*, p. 305.

60D
TRUE—The medial wall of the orbit is formed, from posterior to anterior, by the body of the sphenoid, the orbital plate of the ethmoid, the lacrimal bone and the frontal process of the maxilla. In the orbit, the ethmoid articulates with the maxilla, forming part of the floor, and with the orbital process of the palatine bone. Reference *H*, p. 219 (Fig. 6-5).

60E
TRUE—The superior and middle conchae are part of the ethmoid bone and form part of the lateral wall of the nasal cavity. Reference *H*, p. 289.

61 The maxillary antra:

A. Are aerated at birth.
B. Extend into the zygomatic process of the maxilla.
C. May normally have a small fluid level in the erect position.
D. Have the molar and second premolar teeth usually embedded in the floor.
E. Are best demonstrated on plain radiographs by the PA projection with the base line parallel to the central ray.

62 In the normal skull:

A. The frontal sinuses may extend into the orbital plate of the frontal bone.
B. The average basal angle is about 115 degrees.
C. Habenular calcification is seen posterior to the pineal.
D. Habenular calcification occurs in the habenular commissure.
E. The impressions due to arachnoid granulations are most frequently seen in the squamous temporal bones.

Answers overleaf

61A
FALSE—They are small and contain myxomatous tissue at birth. Reference *H*, p. 292.

61B
TRUE—Reference *G*, p. 320.

61C
FALSE—This is abnormal and may be seen in sinusitis. Reference *H*, p. 293.

61D
TRUE—Reference *H*, p. 292.

61E
FALSE—The best projection is that of Water's which is an occipitomental with the base line at 45 degrees to the central ray. The submentovertical provides a supplementary view. Reference *H*, p. 294.

62A
TRUE—In this situation, a fracture of the frontal bone may lead to air being introduced into the orbital soft tissues. Reference *H*, p. 294.

62B
FALSE—The basal angle is that between a line drawn from the root of the nose to the planum sphenoidale and a line drawn along the slope of the clivus. Its average measurement is 137 degrees. Reference *H*, p. 243.

62C
FALSE—It forms a C-shaped area of calcification anterior to the pineal on a lateral radiograph. Reference *H*, p. 245 (Fig. 6-32B).

62D
FALSE—It occurs in the choroid plexus of the third ventricle. It is separated from the pineal by the commissure. Reference *H*, p. 249.

62E
FALSE—They are most often seen in the parasagittal region adjoining the superior sagittal sinus. Reference *H*, p. 221.

63 The cavernous sinus is related to the:

A. Facial nerve.
B. Sphenoidal air sinus.
C. Diaphragma sella.
D. Sensory ganglion of the trigeminal nerve.
E. Pia mater.

64 The cavernous sinus:

A. Drains into the superior and inferior petrosal sinuses.
B. Is connected to the pterygoid venous plexus via emissary veins.
C. Has the three divisions of the trigeminal nerve in its lateral wall.
D. Receives the occipital sinus.
E. Lies entirely superior to the pituitary gland.

Answers overleaf

63A
FALSE—The nerve has a complex path through the petrous temporal bone before leaving the skull through the stylomastoid foramen. It is not related to the sinus. Reference *G*, p. 354.

63B
TRUE—Reference *H*, p. 295.

63C
TRUE—This is the fold of dura mater which covers the pituitary fossa (Reference *H*, p. 344). It is continuous with the roof of the cavernous sinus (Reference *G*, p. 434).

63D
TRUE—A posterior relation. Reference *G*, p. 434.

63E
FALSE—The cranial venous sinuses lie between layers of dura mater. Reference *G*, p. 432.

64A
TRUE—The superior petrosal sinus joins cavernous and transverse sinuses. The inferior petrosal sinus joins the cavernous sinus to the internal jugular vein. Reference *H*, p. 352.

64B
TRUE—Reference *G*, p. 435.

64C
FALSE—It has the ophthalmic and maxillary divisions only. Reference *G*, p. 434.

64D
FALSE—This small sinus runs from the posterior margin of the foramen magnum to the sinus confluens. It lies in the line of attachment of the falx cerebri to the occipital bone. Reference *H*, p. 467.

64E
FALSE—The cavernous sinus lies to each side of the pituitary. Reference *G*, p. 434.

65 The following are tributaries of the internal jugular vein:

A. The facial vein.
B. The cephalic vein.
C. The posterior auricular vein.
D. The anterior jugular vein.
E. The external jugular vein.

66 The following may be seen on a lateral projection of the skull:

A. The soft palate.
B. The sphenoid air sinus.
C. The lateral mass of the atlas.
D. The frontal sinus.
E. The coronoid process of the mandible.

Answers overleaf

65A
TRUE—This vein forms at the medial angle of the eye and joins the anterior branch of the retromandibular vein. Reference *G*, p. 370.

65B
FALSE—This vein passes along the lateral aspect of the arm and joins the axillary vein after piercing the clavipectoral fascia. Reference *G*, p. 234.

65C
FALSE—This joins the posterior division of the retromandibular vein to form the external jugular. Reference *G*, p. 371.

65D
FALSE—This drains into the external jugular behind the clavicle. Reference *G*, p. 372.

65E
FALSE—This enters the subclavian vein. Reference *G*, p. 372.

66A
TRUE—Reference *H*, p. 268 (Fig. 6-45).

66B
TRUE—Reference *H*, p. 268 (Fig. 6-45).

66C
FALSE—This may be seen on the straight PA view. Reference *H*, p. 266 (Fig. 6-43).

66D
TRUE—Reference *H*, p. 268 (Fig. 6-45).

66E
TRUE—Because it may be superimposed on the inferior turbinate, the coronoid process may simulate a tumour of the maxillary antrum. Reference *X*, p. 136 (Fig. 2-28).

67 The following structures may be identified in the lateral oblique projection of the mastoid process:

- **A.** The mastoid emissary vein.
- **B.** The jugular foramen.
- **C.** The middle ear ossicles.
- →**D.** The cochlea.
- **E.** The styloid process.

68 The following structures may be seen on a standard axial view of the skull:

- **A.** The foramen ovale.
- **B.** The foramen spinosum.
- **C.** The clivus.
- **D.** The nasal septum.
- →**E.** The dorsum sellae.

Answers overleaf

67A
TRUE—This may be seen immediately posterior to the pneumatized portion of the temporal bone. Reference *H*, p. 330.

67B
FALSE—Reference *H*, p. 330.

67C
TRUE—Reference *H*, p. 330.

67D
FALSE—Reference *H*, p. 330.

67E
TRUE—Reference *H*, p. 330.

68A
TRUE—Reference *H*, p. 269 (Fig. 6-46).

68B
TRUE—Reference *H*, p. 269 (Fig. 6-46).

68C
TRUE—Reference *H*, p. 269 (Fig. 6-46).

68D
TRUE—Reference *H*, p. 269 (Fig. 6-46).

68E
FALSE—This is seen on lateral or frontal views of the skull.

69 In the submentovertical (axial) projection of the skull:

A. The cribriform plate is seen.
B. The pharyngeal recess (fossa of Rosenmüller) may be seen.
C. The uvula may be identified as a nodular structure surrounded by air.
D. The zygomatic arch is best seen with a lower kVp exposure.
E. The lateral wall of the maxillary antrum forms a straight line superimposed on the lateral wall of the orbit.

70 The following may be seen on a 30 degrees fronto-occipital (Towne's) projection of the skull:

A. The arcuate eminence.
B. The internal auditory canal.
C. The superior orbital fissure.
D. The head of the mandible.
E. The lesser wing of the sphenoid.

Answers overleaf

69A
FALSE—The hard palate and mandible are superimposed on the medial part of the anterior cranial fossa. (Reference *H*, p. 269 (Fig. 6-46)). As a general rule, the cribriform plate is too thin a structure to cast an image on plain films.

69B
TRUE—Reference *H*, p. 583 (Fig. 10-1 D-F).

69C
TRUE—Reference *H*, p. 581.

69D
TRUE—It tends to be blacked out on the standard film. Reference *H*, p. 276.

69E
FALSE—The antral line is S-shaped, being concave laterally in its anterior portion and convex laterally in its posterior portion. It is superimposed on the straight line formed by the lateral wall of the orbit. Reference *H*, p. 304 (Fig. 7-17B and C).

70A
TRUE—Reference *H*, p. 267 (Fig. 6-44).

70B
TRUE—Reference *H*, p. 267.

70C
FALSE—This is seen on a PA with 15 degrees of caudal tilt of the tube. Reference *H*, p. 265 (Fig. 6-42).

70D
TRUE—Reference *H*, p. 267 (Fig. 6-44).

70E
FALSE—Seen on the PA 15. Reference *H*, p. 265 (Fig. 6-42).

71 Concerning the foramina in the base of the skull:

A. The foramen rotundum is seen on the Towne's projection.
B. The foramen ovale transmits the mandibular nerve.
C. The foramen spinosum transmits the middle cerebral artery.
D. The carotid canal lies posterior to the cochlea.
E. The right jugular foramen is usually larger than the left.

72 The superior orbital fissure:

A. Lies in the greater wing of the sphenoid.
B. Transmits the abducent nerve.
C. Transmits the superior ophthalmic vein.
D. Transmits the ophthalmic artery.
E. Transmits the zygomatic nerve.

Answers overleaf

71A
FALSE—It is seen on PA projections e.g. the PA view with 15 degrees of caudal tube tilt (Caldwell's projection). Reference *H*, p. 236.

71B
TRUE—Reference *H*, p. 241.

71C
FALSE—It transmits the middle meningeal artery. Reference *H*, p. 237.

71D
FALSE—It lies anterior to the cochlea. Reference *H*, p. 239.

71E
TRUE—In 70–90% of cases. Reference *H*, p. 240. This reflects the fact that the right transverse sinus receives the superior sagittal sinus.

72A
FALSE—It lies between the lesser and greater wings of the sphenoid. Reference *G*, p. 312.

72B
TRUE—Reference *G*, p. 312.

72C
TRUE—Reference *G*, p. 312.

72D
FALSE—This accompanies the optic nerve in the optic canal. Reference *G*, p. 312.

72E
FALSE—This passes with the maxillary nerve and a number of communicating veins through the inferior orbital fissure. Reference *G*, p. 312.

73 Relating to the aortic arch and its branches:

A. The common carotid arteries arise from the innominate in about 5% of cases.
B. The common carotid artery usually bifurcates at the level of C2.
C. The left vertebral artery arises directly from the arch in about 4% of cases.
D. The right vertebral artery arises from the right subclavian in less than 50% of cases.
E. An anomalous right subclavian occurs in about 1% of the population.

74 The following arteries arise directly from the external carotid artery:

A. The middle meningeal artery.
B. The maxillary artery.
C. The ascending pharyngeal artery.
D. The ophthalmic artery.
E. The superior thyroid artery.

Answers overleaf

73A
FALSE—This arrangement, which is seen in about 27% of cases, reduces the number of stems arising from the arch to two. Reference *H*, p. 414 (Fig. 8-60).

73B
FALSE—Although the point of bifurcation is variable, it is usual for it to occur at the level of C4. Reference *H*, p. 410.

73C
TRUE—Reference *H*, p. 414 (Fig. 8-60).

73D
FALSE—This occurs in approximately 90% of cases. Reference *H*, p. 446 (Fig. 8-82).

73E
TRUE—Reference *H*, p. 414 (Fig. 8-60).

74A
FALSE—This arises from the maxillary artery. Reference *G*, p. 369.

74B
TRUE—This arises posterior to the neck of the mandible as the larger terminal branch of the external carotid artery. It traverses the infratemporal and pterygopalatine fossae. Reference *G*, p. 369.

74C
TRUE—Reference *G*, p. 368.

74D
FALSE—This is a branch of the internal carotid. Reference *G*, p. 370.

74E
TRUE—It supplies the larynx, the pharynx, the thyroid gland and the infrahyoid muscles. Reference *G*, p. 368.

75 The vertebral artery:

A. Usually arises lateral to the thyrocervical trunk.
B. Passes through the foramen transversarium of C7.
C. Is related to the lateral edge of the posterior atlanto-occipital membrane.
D. Is not related to the vertebral veins.
E. Supplies the spinal cord.

76 The subclavian artery:

A. Gives rise to the internal mammary artery.
B. Gives off the acromiothoracic artery.
C. Lies posterior to scalenus anterior.
D. Gives rise to the inferior thyroid artery via the thyrocervical trunk.
E. May enlarge the shadow of the superior mediastinum of normal elderly patients seen on the frontal chest film.

Answers overleaf

75A
FALSE—The vertebral artery is usually the first branch of the subclavian. Reference *H*, p. 445.

75B
FALSE—It passes through the foramen transversarium of the upper six cervical vertebrae. Reference *H*, p. 445.

75C
TRUE—Reference *P*3, p. 142. Some of the lateral fibres of the membrane may ossify. This may produce the appearance of a foramen on the lateral view of the neck; the so-called arcuate foramen. Reference *X*, p. 168 (Fig. 3-20).

75D
FALSE—As it passes through the foramina transversaria of the cervical vertebrae, the artery is accompanied by one or two vertebral veins. Reference *P*3, p. 138.

75E
TRUE—Through branches in the neck and via the anterior spinal artery. Reference *G*, p. 435.

76A
TRUE—Reference *G*, p. 365.

76B
FALSE—This is a branch of the axillary artery. Reference *G*, p. 202.

76C
TRUE—For descriptive purposes, the artery can be divided into three parts: the second part lies behind scalenus anterior, the first part lies medial to it, and the third part extends lateral to it. Reference *P*3, p. 114.

76D
TRUE—Reference *G*, p. 367.

76E
TRUE—Reference *X*, p. 719 (Fig. 9-155).

77 Concerning variations in the arterial circle of Willis:

A. The presence of all its components with normal diameters is found in a minority of cases.
B. The posterior communicating artery may normally have a funnel-shaped appearance in its proximal portion.
C. The vertebral arteries are usually the same size.
D. A trigeminal artery may be rarely present.
E. Lateral displacement of the basilar artery is a finding that usually signifies a mass lesion.

78 The internal carotid artery:

A. Gives rise to the posterior communicating artery.
B. Passes through the cavernous sinus.
C. Passes to the lateral side of the anterior clinoid process.
D. Gives off the meningo-hypophyseal artery.
E. May give rise to the anterior choroidal artery.

Answers overleaf

77A
TRUE—In 18% of individuals only. Reference *H*, p. 461.

77B
TRUE—The funnel, which is called an infundibulum, should not be confused with an aneurysm. Reference *H*, p. 434 (Fig. 8-74).

77C
FALSE—In only 25% of cases. Reference *H*, p. 463.

77D
TRUE—This forms a carotid–basilar channel as a result of persistence of an embryonic vessel into adult life. Reference *H*, p. 448 (Fig. 8-83).

77E
FALSE—Although it is usually in the midline, it may normally deviate considerably, especially in older individuals. Reference *H*, p. 445.

78A
TRUE—This is given off in the chiasmatic cistern. Reference *H*, p. 424.

78B
TRUE—Crossed on its lateral side by the abducent nerve. Reference *G*, p. 370.

78C
FALSE—It passes to the medial side. Reference *G*, p. 370.

78D
TRUE—This artery is given off within the cavernous sinus. Reference *H*, p. 422.

78E
TRUE—It is given off in the region of the bifurcation into anterior and middle cerebral arteries. Reference *H*, p. 426.

79 The anterior cerebral artery gives off:

A. The anterior communicating artery.
B. The frontopolar artery.
C. Temporal branches.
D. The pericallosal artery.
E. A callosomarginal branch.

80 The middle cerebral artery:

A. Is smaller than the anterior cerebral artery.
B. Passes into the lateral sulcus.
C. Gives off the posterior choroidal arteries.
D. Gives off the posterior temporal artery.
E. Supplies the central and precentral gyri.

Answers overleaf

79A

TRUE—This connects the two anterior cerebral arteries immediately anterior to the lamina terminalis. Reference *H*, p. 433.

79B

TRUE—Reference *H*, p. 432 (Fig. 8-73).

79C

FALSE—Reference *H*, p. 432 (Fig. 8-73).

79D

TRUE—Reference *H*, p. 432 (Fig. 8-73).

79E

TRUE—Reference *H*, p. 432 (Fig. 8-73). The principal arteries deriving their origin from the anterior cerebral artery are the anterior striate, the frontobasal, the frontopolar, the callosomarginal, the pericallosal and the posterior frontal (in that order). The anterior striate arteries are given off before the anterior communicating artery.

80A

FALSE—The middle cerebral artery is the largest branch of the internal carotid. Reference *H*, p. 437.

80B

TRUE—Reference *G*, p. 430.

80C

FALSE—These are derived from the posterior cerebral artery. Reference *H*, p. 458.

80D

TRUE—Reference *H*, p. 438 (Fig. 8-77).

80E

TRUE—Via the precentral and central arteries which frequently have a common trunk. Reference *H*, p. 438 (Fig. 8-77).

81 Concerning the blood supply of the posterior cranial fossa:

A. The basilar artery lies anterior to the pons.
B. The basilar artery cannot be seen on a CT scan without contrast enhancement.
C. The posterior inferior cerebellar artery is usually a branch of the basilar.
D. The posterior cerebral artery may derive its blood supply from either the internal carotid or vertebral systems.
E. The internal auditory artery is a branch of the posterior cerebral.

82 Intracranial calcification may normally occur in the:

A. Petroclinoid ligaments.
B. Falx cerebri.
C. Anterior commissure.
D. Temporal lobes.
E. Basal ganglia.

Answers overleaf

81A
TRUE—Reference *H*, p. 455.

81B
FALSE—It may be seen on a plain scan surrounded by cerebrospinal fluid in the prepontine and basal cisterns.

81C
FALSE—Although it may arise from the basilar artery, it usually arises from the vertebral. Reference *H*, p. 447.

81D
TRUE—This is because the posterior communicating artery arises about 1 cm from the origin of the posterior cerebral and connects it to the internal carotid. Reference *H*, p. 458.

81E
FALSE—It usually arises from the anterior inferior cerebellar artery, but may arise from the basilar. Reference *H*, p. 455.

82A
TRUE—This occurs in about 12% of adults and forms a thin calcific shadow extending posteriorly from the dorsum sella to the petrous ridge. It may be demonstrated in lateral or frontal projection. Reference *H*, p. 250.

82B
TRUE—This occurs in about 7% of adults. Reference *H*, p. 249.

82C
FALSE

82D
FALSE

82E
TRUE—This may be visible on the plain film (Reference *H*, p. 251; Fig. 6-34E). It is quite commonly seen on a CT scan.

83 The following structures pass through the foramen magnum:

A. The spinal accessory nerve.
B. The lesser petrosal nerve.
C. The spinal arteries.
D. The vertebral arteries.
E. The glossopharyngeal nerve.

84 The following are directly related to the lateral ventricles:

A. The septum pellucidum.
B. The hippocampus.
C. The claustrum.
D. The corpus callosum.
E. The trochlear nerve nucleus.

Answers overleaf

83A
TRUE—Reference *H*, p. 242.

83B
FALSE—This goes through the foramen ovale (Reference *G*, p. 348). It conveys parasympathetic fibres from the otic ganglion to the parotid gland Reference *G*, p. 375.

83C
TRUE—Reference *H*, p. 242.

83D
TRUE—Reference *H*, p. 242.

83E
FALSE—This passes through the jugular foramen. Reference *H*, p. 240.

84A
TRUE—It forms the medial wall of the body and anterior horn. Reference *H*, p. 379.

84B
TRUE—It forms the floor of the inferior horn. Reference *H*, p. 379.

84C
FALSE—The claustrum is a thin sheet of grey matter lying deep to the insula. It is not related to the lateral ventricles. Reference *G*, p. 390 (Fig. 32-5).

84D
TRUE—It forms the roof of the body and anterior horn, and one of the walls of the occipital horn and trigone. Reference *H*, p. 379.

84E
FALSE—This lies in the peri-aqueductal grey matter. Reference *G*, p. 350.

85 The third ventricle:

A. Lies between the thalami.
B. Communicates with the lateral ventricles through the interventricular foramina.
C. Is related to the infundibulum of the pituitary.
D. Has the facial colliculus in its floor.
E. Has the optic chiasm in its floor.

86 The following are direct relations of the third ventricle:

A. The massa intermedia (interthalamic connection).
B. The superior medullary velum.
C. The globus pallidus.
D. The posterior commissure.
E. The column of the fornix.

Answers overleaf

85A
TRUE—They form the lateral walls of the ventricle. Reference *H*, p. 382.

85B
TRUE—The foramina are located anterosuperiorly. Reference *H*, p. 381.

85C
TRUE—The infundibular recess forms part of the floor of the ventricle. Reference *H*, p. 382.

85D
FALSE—This lies on the floor of the fourth ventricle, above the striae medullares. Reference *G*, p. 412.

85E
TRUE—Reference *H*, p. 382.

86A
TRUE—This structure bridges the third ventricle between the thalami. Reference *H*, p. 373 (Fig. 8-19A).

86B
FALSE—This is a glial sheet in the roof of the fourth ventricle which stretches between the superior cerebellar peduncles (brachium conjunctivi). Reference *H*, p. 373 (Fig. 8-19A).

86C
FALSE—This is the medial part of the lentiform nucleus and is separated from the third ventricle by the genu of the internal capsule, to which it is directly related, and by the thalamus. Reference *G*, p. 390 (Fig. 32-5).

86D
TRUE—This structure lies in its posterior wall. Reference *H*, p. 373 (Fig. 8-19A).

86E
TRUE—This forms a ridge in the anterolateral wall of the ventricle and lies immediately anterior to, and partly hides, the interventricular foramen. Reference *H*, p. 373 (Fig. 8-19A).

87 The cerebral aqueduct of Sylvius is directly related to:

A. The tectum of the midbrain (the quadrigeminal plate).
B. The lamina terminalis.
C. The tegmentum of the midbrain.
D. The oculomotor nucleus.
E. The mammillary bodies.

88 In the fourth ventricle:

A. The angle between the superior and inferior medullary vela is known as the iter.
B. There is a foramen in each lateral recess which communicates with the subarachnoid space.
C. The pineal is a direct anterior relation.
D. The vagal triangle is situated to either side of the median sulcus in the ventricular floor.
E. The pulvinar forms a ridge in the floor.

Answers overleaf

87A
TRUE—A posterior relation. Reference *H*, p. 373 (Fig. 8-19A).

87B
FALSE—This forms the main anterior boundary to the third ventricle. Reference *H*, p. 373 (Fig. 8-19A).

87C
TRUE—This lies anteriorly. Reference *G*, p. 401.

87D
TRUE—Reference *G*, p. 401.

87E
FALSE—Part of the floor of the third ventricle is formed by the mammillary bodies. Reference *H*, p. 373 (Fig. 8-19A).

88A
FALSE—The iter is the opening of the aqueduct into the third ventricle. The angle between the vela is known as the fastigium. Reference *H*, p. 387.

88B
TRUE—Reference *G*, p. 411. These are known as the foramina of Luschka.

88C
FALSE—The pineal is a posterior relation of the third ventricle. Reference *H*, p. 373 (Fig. 8-19A).

88D
TRUE—Below the striae medullares. Reference *G*, p. 400 (Fig. 33-1).

88E
FALSE—The pulvinar is the wide posterior part of the thalamus. Reference *G*, p. 392.

89 The ambient cistern:

A. Connects the interpeduncular and quadrigeminal cisterns.
B. Contains the anterior cerebral artery.
C. Contains the anterior and posterior choroidal arteries.
D. Contains the posterior cerebral artery.
E. Cannot be identified at computed tomography (CT).

90 The quadrigeminal cistern contains:

A. The inferior sagittal sinus.
B. The great vein of Galen.
C. The posterior cerebral arteries.
D. The distal portion of the medial posterior choroidal artery.
E. The bifurcation of the basilar artery.

Answers overleaf

89A
TRUE—Reference *H*, p. 356 (Fig. 8-6).

89B
FALSE—The artery passes towards the midline and superiorly over the anterior part of the corpus callosum. Reference *G*, p. 429.

89C
TRUE—Reference *H*, p. 365 (Table 8-4).

89D
TRUE—The basal vein and superior cerebellar artery are also contained within the cistern. Reference *H*, p. 365 (Table 8-4).

89E
FALSE—It is readily identifiable. Reference *H*, (Appendix A, p. xii).

90A
FALSE—This is contained within the free inferior edge of the falx cerebri. Reference *H*, p. 350.

90B
TRUE—Reference *H*, p. 365 (Table 8-4).

90C
FALSE—These arteries encircle the brain stem within the ambient cistern. In the distal part of their course, they approach the quadrigeminal cistern without entering it. Reference *H*, p. 458.

90D
TRUE—Reference *H*, p. 365 (Table 8-4).

90E
FALSE—This usually occurs at the level of the dorsum sellae in the interpeduncular cistern. Reference *H*, p. 455.

91 Concerning vascular impressions on the bony cranium:

A. Arteries cannot be distinguished from veins.
B. They tend to be more angular than fractures.
C. Their tendency to occur in characteristic locations is an important feature in distinguishing them from fractures.
D. There is an anastomosis between the middle meningeal artery and a meningeal branch of the ophthalmic artery.
E. The groove due to the middle meningeal vessels normally measures 5 mm in width.

92 Concerning the sutures of the skull:

A. The sagittal and coronal sutures meet at the pterion.
B. The lambda marks the point where the coronal suture meets the sphenoid bone.
C. The lambdoid and squamosal sutures meet at the asterion.
D. A wormian bone is a sutural bone existing within a suture.
E. Sutural sclerosis is a normal process.

Answers overleaf

91A

FALSE—It may be possible to distinguish them apart by the tendency of arteries to taper progressively as they ascend and of veins to maintain a constant width. Reference *H*, p. 222.

91B

FALSE—Vascular impressions are usually more smooth and undulating in their course than the generally angular fractures. Reference *H*, p. 222.

91C

TRUE—Reference *H*, p. 222.

91D

TRUE—This is an anastomosis between branches of the internal and external carotid arteries. Reference *H*, p. 224 (Fig. 6-11C).

91E

FALSE—The average width is 1.5 mm with a maximum normal width of 2 mm. Reference *H*, p. 226.

92A

FALSE—This is the bregma. Reference *H*, p. 227.

92B

FALSE—This is the pterion. Reference *H*, p. 227.

92C

TRUE—Reference *H*, p. 227.

92D

TRUE—Named after Olaus Worms, a Dane. Reference *H*, p. 231.

92E

TRUE—The sclerosis occurs as the result of a bridging process across the suture. It becomes more apparent with advancing age. Reference *H*, p. 232.

93 The hypoglossal canal:

A. Transmits the occipital artery.
B. Transmits a meningeal branch of the ascending pharyngeal artery.
C. May be seen on a submentovertical projection.
D. Is seen on the Stenver's view.
E. May normally measure up to 11 mm in diameter.

94 The following produce vascular impressions which may be seen normally on a lateral film of the skull:

A. The superficial temporal artery.
B. The posterior division of the middle meningeal vessels.
C. The posterior auricular artery.
D. The lateral (sigmoid) sinus.
E. The supra-orbital artery.

Answers overleaf

93A

FALSE—The occipital artery, which arises opposite the facial artery, passes backwards medial to the mastoid process and upwards over the posterior aspect of the skull. Reference *G*, p. 369.

93B

TRUE—Reference *H*, p. 339. This branch may anastomose with the posterior branch of the middle meningeal artery. Reference *H*, p. 224 (Fig. 6-11C).

93C

FALSE—Reference *H*, p. 339.

93D

TRUE—The hypoglossal canals lie on or very near a line joining the external auditory canals, and are therefore seen on oblique views of the skull which place their axis perpendicular to the beam, e.g. the Stenver's. The canal is seen as a ring. Reference *H*, p. 339.

93E

TRUE—Reference *H*, p. 343.

94A

TRUE—The middle temporal branch forms a vertically orientated line on the outer table of the squamous temporal bone anterior to and extending above the external auditory meatus. Reference *H*, p. 222.

94B

TRUE—These anastomose with the branches of the ascending pharyngeal vessels. Reference *H*, p. 224 (Fig. 6-11E).

94C

FALSE—It does not form a visible impression. This branch of the external carotid runs over the mastoid process supplying the parotid gland.

94D

TRUE—Reference *H*, p. 224 (Fig. 6-11E).

94E

TRUE—Reference *H*, p. 224 (Fig. 6-11E).

95 Relating to cerebral veins and venous sinuses:

A. The superior sagittal sinus usually drains into the right transverse sinus.
B. The superior petrosal sinus passes through the jugular foramen.
C. The confluence of sinuses usually lies about 5 cm above the internal occipital protuberance.
D. The basal vein usually drains into the occipital sinus.
E. The internal cerebral veins form at the confluence of septal and thalamostriate veins.

96 There are direct communications between:

A. The mastoid emissary veins and the sigmoid sinuses.
B. The inferior sagittal and straight sinuses.
C. The great vein of Galen and the superior sagittal sinus.
D. The occipital and superior petrosal sinuses.
E. The sphenoparietal and cavernous sinuses.

Answers overleaf

95A
TRUE—Reference *H*, p. 350. Hence, the right sinus is usually larger than the left.

95B
FALSE—This sinus is situated along the superior border of the petrous bone in the attachment of the tentorium cerebelli, and drains into the transverse sinus (Reference *H*, p. 352). The inferior petrosal sinus passes through the jugular foramen Reference *H*, p. 240.

95C
FALSE—The confluence occurs opposite to the protuberance. Reference *H*, p. 352.

95D
FALSE—It usually drains into the great cerebral vein of Galen. Reference *H*, p. 475.

95E
TRUE—Reference *H*, p. 470.

96A
TRUE—Reference *H*, p. 227.

96B
TRUE—The inferior sagittal sinus lies in the free inferior edge of the falx and ends in the straight sinus. Reference *H*, p. 352.

96C
FALSE—The internal cerebral veins unite to form the great vein, which then enters the inferior sagittal sinus. Reference *H*, p. 474.

96D
FALSE—The occipital sinus drains into the sinus confluens. The superior petrosal sinus join the cavernous and transverse sinuses. Reference *H*, p. 352.

96E
TRUE—The sphenoparietal sinus begins just posterior to the coronal suture and courses along the lesser wing of the sphenoid to enter the cavernous sinus. Reference *H*, p. 227.

97 In the vertebral column:

A. The nucleus pulposus represents a persistence of the notochord into adulthood.
B. Secondary ossification centres appear in the second year of life.
C. The secondary ossification centres are situated in the laminae.
D. A narrow L5–S1 joint space may be normal.
E. A sagittal diameter of 15 mm or less in the cervical spinal canal is abnormal.

98 In the spinal canal:

A. The cord is suspended by the anterior and posterior longitudinal ligaments.
B. The cord has its widest diameter at C3.
C. The artery of Adamkiewicz (arterioradicularis magna) is derived directly from the vertebral artery.
D. The anterior spinal artery may be seen normally at myelography.
E. The cord usually ends at the level of the third lumbar vertebra.

Answers overleaf

97A
TRUE—Reference *H*, p. 514.

97B
FALSE—They appear at puberty. Reference *H*, p. 517.

97C
FALSE—They appear at the tips of the spinous and transverse processes and at the upper and lower surfaces of the vertebral body. Reference *H*, p. 517.

97D
TRUE—At this point there is the junction of the lumbar and sacral curves. When narrowing occurs in the absence of other changes, it should be considered a normal finding. Reference *H*, p. 517.

97E
FALSE—A measurement of 10 mm or less is likely to be associated with cord compression. Reference *H*, p. 534.

98A
FALSE—The lateral ligaments of the cord, the denticulate ligaments, do this. Reference *H*, p. 565.

98B
FALSE—It is widest at C5 where the diameter is normally 12–14 mm. It is also enlarged at the level of T12 where it normally measures 11–13 mm in diameter. Reference *H*, p. 565.

98C
FALSE—It is derived from the anterior radicular branch of one of the larger segmental arteries in the region of T8 to L4. In about 60% of people, it is left sided. It is the major segmental arterial supply to the dorsolumbar spine and anastomoses with the anterior spinal artery. Reference *H*, p. 575.

98D
TRUE—It produces a vertical, linear, midline filling-defect. This should not be confused with the tortuous, dilated vessels of a spinal angioma. Reference *E*, p. 1120.

98E
FALSE—It usually ends at the L1–2 interspace. Reference *H*, p. 565.

99 In the vertebral column:

A. The bony union of the neural arch begins in the sacral region.
B. The anterior margin of C5 may normally be narrowed compared with the posterior margin.
C. 'Schmorl's nodes' are central notches in the surfaces of bodies of thoracic vertebrae.
D. Extra apophyses occur along the postero-superior surface of the bodies of lumbar vertebrae.
E. The ligamentum flavum is part of the anterior boundary of the spinal canal.

100 The shoulder joint:

A. Has a dependent pouch in the axillary part of the joint capsule.
B. Usually communicates with the subscapular bursa.
C. Usually communicates with the subacromial bursa.
D. Encloses the short head of biceps.
E. Is related to the axillary nerve.

Answers overleaf

99A
FALSE—It begins in the neck at about the age of 3, and proceeds caudally to the sacrum which starts to ossify at 6–7 years. Reference *H*, p. 521.

99B
TRUE—And, less commonly, this infantile configuration may also persist in C6. It should not be interpreted as compression. Reference *H*, p. 538.

99C
TRUE—Their frequent occurrence in adults (about 40%) has made their significance debatable. Reference *H*, p. 544.

99D
FALSE—They occur along the antero-superior surface. Reference *H*, p. 518. (Fig. 9-12).

99E
FALSE—It lies posteriorly, uniting the laminae of adjacent vertebrae. Reference *H*, p. 562.

100A
TRUE—Reference *H*, p. 80 (Fig. 4-15B and C). This is because the capsule is lax and because it extends inferiorly onto the surgical neck of the humerus.

100B
TRUE—Reference *G*, p. 195. The bursa lies deep to the subscapularis muscle, anterior to the joint and inferior to the coracoid process.

100C
FALSE—Although it may rarely do so. Reference *P*1, p. 78.

100D
FALSE—The long head passes in a tubular sheath of synovium through the joint. This sheath is prolonged under the transverse humeral ligament into the intertubercular groove. The long head is attached to the supraglenoid tubercle. Reference *G*, p. 204.

100E
TRUE—It is related inferiorly to the axillary nerve. Reference *G*, p. 195.

101 The axillary artery:

A. Gives off the suprascapular artery.
B. Supplies the female breast via the medial thoracic artery.
C. Gives off the posterior humeral circumflex artery.
D. Lies lateral to the axillary vein.
E. Is surrounded by the cords and branches of the brachial plexus.

102 Concerning the arteries in the upper limb:

A. The axillary artery becomes the brachial artery at the outer border of pectoralis minor.
B. The nutrient artery to the humerus is directed proximally towards the shoulder.
C. The brachial artery accompanies the radial nerve in the radial groove.
D. The brachial artery may divide into radial and ulnar branches opposite the mid-humerus.
E. The deep palmar arch is given off distal to the superficial arch.

Answers overleaf

101A
FALSE—This is derived from the thyrocervical trunk. Reference *G*, p. 367.

101B
FALSE—The main branch of the axillary artery supplying the breast is the lateral thoracic. Reference *G*, p. 202.

101C
TRUE—This is the larger of the humeral circumflex arteries. Reference *P*1, p. 29.

101D
TRUE—The vein lies medially and overlaps the artery anteriorly. As the arm is abducted, the vein comes to lie more and more anteriorly. Reference *P*1, p. 29.

101E
TRUE—Reference *G*, p. 201. The nerves may be compressed by haematoma when the artery is punctured at angiography.

102A
FALSE—This occurs at the outer border of teres major. The anterior wall of the axilla, consisting of the pectoral muscles, extends less distally than the posterior wall, formed laterally by teres major. This leaves the artery covered in its lower third by skin and fascia only (Reference *P*1, p. 27). Hence, one can gain access to the artery for arteriography.

102B
FALSE—It is directed towards the elbow and runs a course of at least 5 cm on the anteromedial border of the humerus. It must not be confused with a fracture. Reference *H*, p. 83.

102C
FALSE—The profunda brachii artery does this. Reference *G*, p. 205.

102D
TRUE—Reference *H*, p. 85.

102E
FALSE—The opposite occurs. Reference *H*, p. 117 (Fig. 4-45).

103 Concerning normal variation:

A. The paraglenoid fossa is an indentation in the neck of the scapula.
B. An articulation may occur between the coracoid process of the scapula and the conoid tubercle of the clavicle.
C. There may be lucency of the greater tuberosity.
D. A posterior 'fat pad' on the lateral view of the elbow may be seen.
E. Fat lines above and below the neck of the femur may be seen.

104 In the wrist:

A. The arteries supplying the scaphoid bone enter in the distal portion.
B. The capitate articulates with the scaphoid.
C. The capitate articulates with the second, third and fourth metacarpals.
D. The lunate articulates with the trapezoid.
E. The pisiform articulates with the hamate.

Answers overleaf

103A
FALSE—It is a notch in the ilium immediately lateral to the inferior margin of the sacroiliac joint caused by the superior gluteal artery as it leaves the pelvis. Reference *H*, p. 127 (Fig. 5-7).

103B
TRUE—Forming a coracoclavicular joint. Reference *H*, p. 65 (Fig. 4-1B).

103C
TRUE—It may be interpreted as a lytic lesion. Reference *H*, p. 83 (Fig. 4-16D).

103D
FALSE—The visibility of a fat plane behind the olecranon fossa is indicative of a joint effusion and a pathological entity such as a fracture or infection. Reference *H*, p. 93.

103E
TRUE—These are often referred to incorrectly as the joint capsule, but are caused by fat related to muscles. Reference *H*, p. 137 (Fig. 5-17F).

104A
TRUE—Hence, when a fracture occurs, there is a risk of avascular necrosis because the proximal portion may become separated from its blood supply. Reference *H*, p. 104.

104B
TRUE—Reference *H*, p. 106 (Fig. 4-33).

104C
TRUE—Reference *H*, p. 106 (Fig. 4-33).

104D
FALSE—Reference *H*, p. 106 (Fig. 4-33).

104E
FALSE—The pisiform articulates with the triquetral. Reference *G*, p. 223.

105 In the wrist, the proximal row of carpal bones includes:

A. The scaphoid.
B. The trapezoid.
C. The capitate.
D. The lunate.
E. The triquetral.

106 The femoral artery:

A. Is directly related to the hip joint.
B. Supplies the skin in the pudendal region.
C. Is lateral to the femoral vein in its passage through the adductor canal.
D. Gives off the descending genicular artery in the adductor canal.
E. Becomes the popliteal artery after piercing adductor longus.

Answers overleaf

105A
TRUE—Reference *G*, p. 223.

105B
FALSE—Reference *G*, p. 223.

105C
FALSE—Reference *G*, p. 223.

105D
TRUE—Reference *G*, p. 223.

105E
TRUE—From lateral to medial, the bones in the proximal row are the scaphoid, lunate and triquetral. Reference *G*, p. 223.

106A
FALSE—It is separated from the joint by the tendon of psoas. Reference *G*, p. 246.

106B
TRUE—Through the external pudendal artery. Reference *H*, p. 193 (Fig. 5-83).

106C
FALSE—It comes to lie anterior to the vein. Reference *G*, p. 255.

106D
TRUE—This branch springs from the femoral artery a short distance above the opening in the adductor magnus. Reference *P*1, p. 148.

106E
FALSE—It becomes the popliteal artery after piercing adductor magnus, about 10 cm above the knee joint. Reference *G*, p. 253.

107 In the leg:

A. The deep femoral (profunda femoris) artery descends medial to the superficial femoral.
B. The deep femoral artery terminates by dividing into lateral and medial circumflex femoral arteries.
C. The popliteal artery divides at the lower border of the popliteus muscle.
D. The anterior tibial artery supplies the tibial nutrient artery.
E. The peroneal artery is a branch of the posterior tibial.

108 Concerning the anatomy of the lymphatics seen at lymphography:

A. The lymphatics do not have valves.
B. The superficial inguinal nodes usually number five or less.
C. The popliteal nodes drain directly to the deep inguinal nodes.
D. The superficial inguinal nodes drain into the deep inguinal group.
E. The superficial inguinal nodes receive lymph from the abdominal wall up to the level of the umbilicus.

Answers overleaf

107A
FALSE—It descends lateral to the superficial femoral. Reference *H*, p. 192 (Fig. 5-82). It arises in the femoral triangle about 4–5 cm below the inguinal ligament.

107B
FALSE—Although these are branches of the deep femoral artery, it terminates by perforating the adductor magnus muscle and dividing into muscular branches. Reference *H*, p. 192.

107C
TRUE—It divides into anterior and posterior tibial arteries. Reference *H*, p. 192.

107D
FALSE—This arises from the posterior tibial artery (Reference *H*, p. 195.) The nutrient foramina in the leg lie on the posterior surfaces and are directed away from the knee. Reference *H*, p. 42 (Fig. 3-6).

107E
TRUE—It arises about 2.5 cm below the distal border of popliteus. Reference *H*, p. 194.

108A
FALSE—The abundant valves confer a beaded appearance to the lymphatics, and prevent backflow. Reference *H*, p. 200.

108B
FALSE—They usually number 10–20. Reference *H*, p. 202.

108C
TRUE—Reference *H*, p. 202.

108D
TRUE—As well as to the lower external iliac nodes. Reference *H*, p. 202.

108E
TRUE—They receive lymph from a large area which also includes the gluteal region, the superficial structures of the legs and the external genitalia. Reference *H*, p. 202.

109 In the hip joint:

A. The capsule is attached to the intertrochanteric line.
B. The capsule is attached to the intertrochanteric crest.
C. The ischio-femoral ligament is one of the strongest in the body.
D. The ilio-femoral ligament is attached to the anterior superior iliac spine.
E. The angle between the axes of the neck and shaft of the femur is normally 100 degrees.

110 Relating to the hips and pelvis:

A. The obturator internis muscle may be seen on films of the pelvis.
B. Adductor magnus is attached to the superior ramus of the pubic bone.
C. The lesser trochanter is well shown in the standard AP view of the hip.
D. In the AP projection, a line drawn along the outer margin of the femoral neck should intersect the femoral head.
E. A double ossification centre for the femoral head is an indication of disease.

Answers overleaf

109A
TRUE—Reference *H*, p. 141 (Fig. 5-23).

109B
FALSE—Reference *H*, p. 141 (Fig. 5-23).

109C
FALSE—It is a weak ligament. The Y-shaped ilio-femoral ligament, however, is one of the strongest, rivalled only by the interosseus ligament of the sacroiliac joint. Reference *P*3, pp. 182–3.

109D
FALSE—It is attached to the anterior inferior iliac spine. Reference *G*, p. 245.

109E
FALSE—It varies between 110 and 140 degrees in the adult, with a mean of 127. The normal angle is greater than this at birth. Reference *H*, p. 134.

110A
TRUE—Reference *X*, p. 843 (Fig. 12-2).

110B
FALSE—It is attached to the inferior ramus and the ischial tuberosity (Reference *P*1, p. 153 (Fig. 105)). The attachment of the adductor magnus muscle may be the site for an avulsion fracture.

110C
FALSE—The lesser trochanter is shown in maximum detail, and the neck of the femur is foreshortened, if the foot is everted. In the positioning for the AP view, the foot is inverted approximately 15 degrees. Reference *H*, p. 148 (Fig. 5-31).

110D
TRUE—In both AP and lateral projections (Reference *H*, p. 137). The femoral head may not be crossed by such a line when a slipped epiphysis is present.

110E
FALSE—It is a normal variant. Reference *X*, p. 444 (Fig. 7-5).

111 Concerning the hip joint:

A. The psoas bursa may communicate with the joint cavity.
B. Shenton's line joins the inferior margin of the obturator foramen to the inferior aspect of the femoral neck.
C. Piriformis is an anterior relation.
D. The ligament of the femoral head (ligamentum teres) carries a small branch of the obturator artery.
E. Gluteus medius lies superiorly.

112 In the knee:

A. The anterior margin of the normal patella is often irregular.
B. The lateral articular surface of the patella is smaller than the medial articular surface.
C. The oblique popliteal ligament is an extension of the semitendinosus muscle.
D. The thickenings of the joint capsule which bind the menisci to the outer margins of the tibia are the triangular ligaments.
E. Part of the blood supply is derived from the descending branch of the lateral femoral circumflex artery.

Answers overleaf

111A
TRUE—This separates the iliopsoas muscle from the superior ramus of the pubic bone. It may communicate with the joint cavity between the iliofemoral and pubofemoral ligaments. Reference *G*, p. 246.

111B
FALSE—The line passes along the superior and medial margins of the obturator foramen, not the inferior margin (Reference *H*, p. 143). This line is used in the evaluation of the joint in cases of trauma.

111C
FALSE—It lies posteriorly with the quadratus femoris, obturator internis, the gemelli, and the inferior gluteal nerve and vessels. Reference *G*, p. 246 (Fig. 21-3).

111D
TRUE—Reference *H*, p. 138.

111E
TRUE—With the reflected head of rectus femoris and the superior gluteal nerve and vessels. Reference *G*, p. 246 (Fig. 21-3).

112A
TRUE—An appearance caused by tendinous insertions and nutrient arteries. It should not be considered pathological. Reference *H*, p. 166.

112B
FALSE—The lateral is the larger. Reference *G*, p. 257.

112C
FALSE—It is an extension of semimembranosus. Reference *G*, p. 260.

112D
FALSE—They are the coronary ligaments. Reference *G*, p. 260.

112E
TRUE—Reference *H*, p. 193.

113 In the knee:

- **A.** A popliteal bursa is usually present.
- **B.** The gastrocnemius bursa opens into the joint capsule.
- **C.** The fabella lies in the lateral head of gastrocnemius.
- **D.** The anterior cruciate ligament is attached to the anterior tibial spine.
- **E.** The lateral meniscus is intimately attached to the fibular collateral ligament.

114 In the ankle and foot:

- **A.** There is overlapping of the tibia and fibula on the standard AP view of the ankle.
- **B.** The epiphyseal line at the base of the 5th metatarsal is transversely orientated.
- **C.** The first metatarsal is the longest of the metatarsals.
- **D.** The midline of the adult foot passes through the centre of the talus and the head of the 3rd metatarsal.
- **E.** The long axis of the first metatarsal is parallel to the midline of the foot.

Answers overleaf

113A
FALSE—A bursa in the popliteal space is found in about 13% of knees. When it becomes inflamed, it is frequently referred to as a 'Baker's cyst'. Reference *H*, p. 154.

113B
TRUE—The bursa is situated in the medial head of the muscle. Reference *G*, p. 265.

113C
TRUE—Reference *H*, p. 138.

113D
FALSE—It is attached to the anterior part of the intercondylar area. It passes superiorly, posteriorly and laterally to the medial aspect of the lateral femoral condyle. Reference *G*, p. 260.

113E
FALSE—The lateral meniscus is separate from the collateral ligament. The medial meniscus, however, is firmly connected to the tibial collateral ligament. Reference *H*, p. 152.

114A
TRUE—However, a clear view of the talotibial joint space is obtained by this projection. A view of the distal tibia and fibula where there is no overlap may be obtained by pointing the foot further medially. Reference *H*, p. 177 (Fig. 5-63).

114B
FALSE—It is obliquely orientated. This contrasts with fractures in this region which tend to be transversely orientated. Reference *H*, p. 180.

114C
FALSE—It is the shortest and thickest. The second metatarsal is the longest. Reference *H*, p. 180.

114D
FALSE—The midline passes through the centre of the calcaneus and the head of the 3rd metatarsal. Reference *H*, p. 186.

114E
FALSE—It forms an angle of 15 degrees to the midline of the foot. A line drawn through the long axis of the first metatarsal also passes through the mid-axis of the talus. Reference *H*, p. 186.

115 In the ankle:

A. Part of the medial (deltoid) ligament is attached to the navicular bone.
B. The calcaneus usually articulates with the navicular.
C. The os vesalianum lies adjacent to the navicular.
D. The lower epiphysis of the fibula unites with the shaft at about the 20th year.
E. A secondary ossification centre appears in the calcaneus in the second year.

116 In the foot and ankle:

A. The great saphenous vein ascends anterior to the medial malleolus.
B. The small saphenous vein passes anterior to the lateral malleolus.
C. The anterior tibial artery becomes the dorsal pedis artery.
D. The posterior tibial artery passes posterior to the lateral malleolus.
E. The middle cuneiform is the largest of the cuneiform bones.

Answers overleaf

115A
TRUE—This extremely strong ligament is attached proximally to the medial malleolus and distally to the body of the talus, the sustentaculum tali, the plantar calcaneonavicular ligament, the neck of the talus and the navicular. Reference *G*, p. 277.

115B
FALSE—However, the plantar calcaneonavicular (spring) ligament passes between them, from the sustentaculum tali to the navicular tuberosity. Reference *G*, p. 279.

115C
FALSE—The os tibiale externum lies adjacent to the navicular. The os vesalianum lies immediately proximal to the base of the 5th metatarsal. Reference *H*, p. 173 (Fig. 5-59).

115D
TRUE—Reference *H*, p. 170.

115E
FALSE—It appears at 8–10 years of age (Reference *H*, p. 176). Sclerosis and fragmentation of this secondary ossification centre may be seen frequently and should not be misinterpreted as abnormal. Reference *X*, p. 571 (Fig. 7-250).

116A
TRUE—Having originated from the medial end of the dorsal venous arch. Reference *G*, p. 285.

116B
FALSE—It passes posterior to it. Reference *G*, p. 286.

116C
TRUE—Reference *H*, p. 195.

116D
FALSE—It passes posterior to the medial malleolus. Reference *H*, p. 195.

116E
FALSE—It is the smallest. Reference *G*, p. 275.

117 Concerning the veins of the lower limb:

A. The great saphenous vein joins the femoral vein in the femoral triangle.
B. The small saphenous vein joins the femoral vein in the adductor canal.
C. There is normally no flow of blood from superficial to deep veins.
D. There are numerous valves in the deep veins.
E. The intra-osseus veins of lower tibia and fibula drain into the superficial veins.

118 The following bones have usually begun to ossify at birth:

A. The glenoid cavity of the scapula.
B. The calcaneus.
C. The scaphoid.
D. The talus.
E. The head of the humerus.

Answers overleaf

117A
TRUE—The great saphenous vein passes through the saphenous opening which is an oval deficiency in the fascia lata. The fascia lata forms the roof of the femoral triangle. The opening is situated about 3 cm inferior and lateral to the pubic tubercle. Reference *G*, p. 253.

117B
FALSE—The small saphenous joins the popliteal vein after piercing the fascial roof of the popliteal fossa. Reference *G*, p. 286.

117C
FALSE—There are communicating branches allowing flow from the superficial to the deep systems (Reference *H*, p. 198C). Valves prevent flow in the opposite direction.

117D
TRUE—They are more numerous than in the superficial veins. Reference *H*, p. 199.

117E
FALSE—The contrast from an intra-osseus injection preferentially fills the deep system. The medullary cavity of the medial malleolus is the larger and is the better site for injection. Reference *L*, p. 47.

118A
FALSE—Although much of the scapula is ossified at birth, the glenoid cavity, the acromion, the coracoid process, the vertebral border and the inferior angle are cartilaginous. Ossification of the glenoid begins at about the age of 10 years. Reference *H*, pp. 66–7.

118B
TRUE—This bone is invariably ossified. The ossification centre appears at about 7 months *in utero*. Reference *G*, p. 273 (Fig. 23-1).

118C
FALSE—The ossification centre for the scaphoid appears at about 4–7 years of age. Reference *H*, p. 59 (Table 3-2).

118D
TRUE—The ossification centre of the talus appears about 1 month after that of the calcaneus. Reference *G*, p. 273 (Fig. 23-1).

118E
TRUE—Reference *H*, p. 59 (Table 3-2).

119 The following have usually begun to ossify at birth:

A. The head of the femur.
B. The lower femoral ossification centre.
C. The lower tibial ossification centre.
D. The navicular bone.
E. The greater tuberosity of the humerus.

120 The following bones have not usually begun to ossify in a 6-year-old child:

A. The patella.
B. The tibial tuberosity.
C. The lateral epicondyle of the elbow.
D. The capitulum of the humerus.
E. The iliac crest.

Answers overleaf

119A
FALSE—This usually begins to ossify in the first 8 months of post-natal life. Reference *H*, p. 59 (Table 3-2).

119B
TRUE—This appears at 8–9 months *in utero*. Reference *G*, p. 243 (Fig. 21-1).

119C
FALSE—This appears at about 1 year of age. Reference *G*, p. 259 (Fig. 22-2).

119D
FALSE—This is usually the last of the tarsal bones to ossify. This generally happens between 2 and 5 years of age. Reference *H*, p. 59 (Table 3-2).

119E
FALSE—This begins to ossify in the first year of life. Reference *H*, p. 59 (Table 3-2).

120A
FALSE—Ossification will normally have occurred by the sixth year. Reference *H*, p. 59 (Table 3-2).

120B
TRUE—Not usually ossified before the tenth to twelfth years. Reference *H*, p. 59 (Table 3-2).

120C
TRUE—Ossifies at about 9–11 years of age. Reference *H*, p. 59 (Table 3-2).

120D
FALSE—Usually ossified by the age of 2. Reference *H*, p. 59 (Table 3-2).

120E
TRUE—The ossification centre for the iliac crest appears at puberty. Reference *H*, p. 59 (Table 3-2).

II. RADIOLOGICAL PHYSICS

RADIOLOGICAL PHYSICS

1 Concerning atoms and their description:

A. The mass number defines the number of nucleons (protons and neutrons).
B. The M shell may contain 20 electrons.
C. Isotopes of an element have different chemical properties.
D. Decay of $^{11}_{6}C$ to $^{11}_{5}B$ involves the emission of a positron.
E. A nuclide can be characterized by its atomic number only.

2 Electromagnetic radiation:

A. Includes infrared light.
B. Includes radio waves.
C. Can behave as a particle.
D. Includes beta emission.
E. Has an energy that is proportional to the wavelength.

Answers overleaf

1A
TRUE—For example, ^{24}Na which is an isotope of sodium containing 24 nuclear particles (protons and neutrons). It is radioactive. Reference *A*, p. 18.

1B
FALSE—It has places for a maximum of 18 electrons. Reference *A*, p. 13.

1C
FALSE—They may have different physical properties. Reference *A*, p. 20.

1D
TRUE—Because a proton has changed into a neutron and lost a unit of positive charge. Reference *C*, p. 9.

1E
FALSE—A nuclide is defined by both atomic number (Z) and mass number (A), and in certain cases by the nuclear energy state. Reference *C*, p. 7.

2A
TRUE—Reference *B*, p. 6.

2B
TRUE—Reference *B*, p. 6.

2C
TRUE—For short-wavelength forms of electromagnetic radiation, such as X-rays. Reference *B*, p. 6.

2D
FALSE

2E
FALSE—The energy is inversely proportional to wavelength, from:

$$E = \frac{hc}{\lambda}$$

where E = energy; h = Planck's constant; c = velocity of light; λ = wavelength. Reference *B*, p. 6.

3 In an X-ray tube:

A. Ceramic envelopes are used.
B. The high atomic number of tungsten favours its use as an anode.
C. The melting point of tungsten is 3380°C.
D. Loss of heat from the housing is chiefly by conduction.
E. Tungsten has a high vapour pressure.

4 In the continuous X-ray spectrum:

A. The quality of the radiation depends on the Z of the target material.
B. The quantity of the radiation is independent of the wave form of the applied voltage.
C. Radiation intensity is proportional to the atomic number of the target material.
D. Radiation quality is independent of tube current.
E. Radiation quantity is proportional to kV^3.

Answers overleaf

3A
FALSE—Borosilicate glass is most often used. Ceramics are used in some tubes to form the bearings for rotating anodes.

3B
TRUE—Because the intensity of radiation emitted from an anode increases in direct proportion to atomic number. Reference *A*, p. 50.

3C
TRUE—It is less likely to melt than other elements that might be used to make an anode. Reference *A*, p. 280.

3D
FALSE—Convection is the chief means of heat loss. Reference *A*, p. 281.

3E
FALSE—It has a low vapour pressure and, therefore, tends not to vaporize. When vaporization occurs, tungsten is deposited on the tube walls and this limits tube life. Reference *A*, p. 280.

4A
FALSE—Quality depends on kVp and wave form only. Reference *A*, p. 49.

4B
FALSE—The wave form influences both the quantity and the quality of the radiation produced. Reference *A*, p. 52.

4C
TRUE—Reference *A*, p. 50.

4D
TRUE—Tube current influences the quantity of radiation produced. Reference *A*, p. 53.

4E
FALSE—It is proportional to kV^2. Reference *A*, p. 51.

7 The spinning top used to measure the length of an exposure from an X-ray tube and single-phase generator:

A. Is motor driven.
B. Has a metal disc with a slit at its edge.
C. Should be rotated at a known velocity.
D. Gives a continuous arc of film exposure.
E. Is able to record variations in tube output.

8 Tube rating:

A. Falls as focal spot size decreases.
B. Falls with time.
C. Increases as exposure time decreases for a tube being used at low kV (less than 40 kV).
D. Increases for exposures of less than 0.02 seconds made with an anode rotating at 3000 rpm.
E. Depends on focal spot size for very long exposures.

Answers overleaf

7A
FALSE—It is manually rotated. Reference *B*, p. 48.

7B
TRUE—Reference *B*, p. 48.

7C
FALSE—The speed of rotation is not important other than that it should be fast enough to separate the pulses and not so fast that it makes a complete revolution during the exposure. Reference *B*, p. 49.

7D
FALSE—This is seen when using a 12-pulse three phase generator. Reference *B*, p. 49.

7E
TRUE—For example, when using a tube from 'cold' or if there is fluctuation in the power supply. With the former example, the slit will expose a smaller area of the film at the beginning of the exposure. Reference *B*, p. 49.

8A
TRUE—Because the heat is spread over a smaller area. Reference *A*, p. 325.

8B
TRUE—Reference *A*, p. 328.

8C
FALSE—It becomes a constant. This is because the tube current depends on filament heating at low kV and there is a limit to this. Reference *A*, p. 321.

8D
FALSE—Because the anode will not have completed a revolution in this time. The focal spot size will be decreased which causes the rating to become constant. Reference *A*, p. 329.

8E
FALSE—It depends on the heat storing and dissipating characteristics of the tube housing. This is the reason why the anode need not be rotated more than very slowly at fluoroscopy. Reference *A*, p. 328.

9 Focal spot size:

A. Is measured with a pin-hole of the same dimensions.
B. Increases with increase in kVp.
C. Increases with increase in mA.
D. Is not affected by radiation distribution when measured with a line-pair resolution test tool.
E. Is measured on the cathode side of the central beam to avoid the heel effect.

10 In an X-ray tube and electric circuit:

A. The stator coils are contained within the glass envelope.
B. Oil is used to lubricate the bearings of a rotating anode.
C. The pre-reading voltmeter indicates the kV of the primary circuit.
D. The ammeter in the secondary coil of the high-tension transformer reads the peak tube current.
E. An electronic timer consists of a capacitor, a variable resistor and a thyratron.

Answers overleaf

9A

FALSE—The pin-hole must be small with respect to the size of the focal spot. This means that very small pin-holes must be used (0.03 mm in diameter) for focal spots below 1 mm in size. Reference *B*, p. 277.

9B

FALSE—A slight decrease is seen. Reference *B*, p. 281.

9C

TRUE—An effect known as focal spot blooming. Reference *B*, p. 281.

9D

FALSE—The measurements obtained are greater than the effective focal spot size (i.e. the actual physical size as determined by a pin-hole camera) when the distribution is of the 'edge band' type; and less when 'centrally peaked' in distribution. Reference *B*, p. 281.

9E

FALSE—All measurements, by whichever method, must be performed in the central axis of the beam. Reference *B*, pp. 277–9.

10A

FALSE—They are situated outside the glass envelope. Reference *A*, p. 288.

10B

FALSE—Being inside a vacuum, a metallic lubricant is required, e.g. lead or silver. Reference *A*, p. 288.

10C

FALSE—It is calibrated to indicate the kV across the tube. Reference *A*, p. 293.

10D

FALSE—It measures the mean current. Reference *A*, p. 299.

10E

TRUE—Reference *B*, p. 45.

11 In the photoelectric effect:

A. 'Free' and 'bound' electrons are equally involved.
B. The mass attenuation coefficient is inversely proportional to Z^3.
C. The mass attenuation coefficient is proportional to the cube of the photon energy.
D. A positron may be emitted.
E. A neutron may be emitted.

12 The photoelectric effect:

A. Occurs more in aluminium than in lead for a given photon energy.
B. Results in the emission of characteristic radiation.
C. Is a pure absorption process in biological materials.
D. Produces scatter radiation.
E. Is most likely to occur when the photon energy and electron binding energy are nearly the same.

Answers overleaf

11A
FALSE—In this phenomenon, a photon disappears on interacting with a bound electron. Reference *A*, p. 69.

11B
FALSE—It is directly proportional to Z^3. Reference *A*, p. 72.

11C
FALSE—It is inversely proportional to the photon energy, so that the process is the dominant attenuation process at low kV. Reference *A*, p. 72.

11D
FALSE—This happens in pair production. Reference *A*, p. 73.

11E
FALSE—This happens at energies in excess of 10 MeV. Reference *A*, p. 73.

12A
FALSE—The number of photoelectric interactions is proportional to Z^3. Lead has the greater Z number (82 compared with 13 for aluminium). Reference *A*, p. 71.

12B
TRUE—This is emitted as electrons fill the vacancies in the k-shell from adjacent shells. Reference *B*, p. 53.

12C
TRUE—Because the characteristic radiation from body materials is of low energy and is absorbed locally. Reference *B*, p. 55.

12D
FALSE—Most scatter in diagnostic radiology is produced by the Compton process. Secondary radiation from the photoelectric effect may reach the film only if it is emitted from high atomic number elements such as barium and iodine. Reference *B*, p. 55.

12E
TRUE—Reference *B*, p. 53.

13 In the Compton effect:

A. The angle of scatter and the energy lost by the photon are related.
B. The amount of scatter is dependent on electron density.
C. The electron density is constant for all elements.
D. Change in wavelength of a scattered photon varies with the Z of the attenuating medium.
E. Scatter is more likely to occur in any direction with increasing photon energy.

14 The following statements are true:

A. Bone absorbs more radiation than muscle when beam energy is low.
B. Absorption of radiation is greater for soft tissue situated near to bone than soft tissue distant from bone.
C. Filters remove high-energy radiation whilst leaving low-energy photons unchanged.
D. A filter attenuates largely by the photoelectric effect.
E. A compound filter consists of several layers of a single element interspaced with a non-attenuating material.

Answers overleaf

13A
TRUE—Reference *A*, p. 65.

13B
TRUE—Because the process involves the interaction of photons and electrons. Reference *A*, p. 66.

13C
FALSE—Hydrogen has about twice the density of electrons of all other elements. Reference *A*, p. 66.

13D
FALSE—The wavelength change depends on angle of scatter only. Reference *A*, p. 66.

13E
FALSE—With increasing energy, the scatter is more likely to occur in a forward direction. Reference *A*, p. 68.

14A
TRUE—Because of the predominance of the photoelectric effect at low kV and in high atomic number elements (Z of bone is 13 and of muscle 7.4). Reference *A*, p. 133.

14B
TRUE—Because of the production of more photoelectrons in bone. Reference *A*, p. 134.

14C
FALSE—Filtration removes the useless low-energy radiation which contributes to the dose without contributing to the image. Reference *B*, p. 78.

14D
TRUE—Reference *B*, p. 78.

14E
FALSE—It consists of two or more layers of different metals. Reference *B*, p. 78.

15 Scatter reaching the film is decreased by:

A. Having a small field size.
B. Decreasing part thickness.
C. Having a large gap between the patient and the film.
D. Placing a filter on the cassette.
E. Placing a filter between the X-ray tube and the patient.

16 In the diagnostic range, increase in the kVp at a constant mAs will:

A. Increase the wavelength of the X-rays emitted.
B. Increase the effect of scatter on the radiograph.
C. Increase the quantity of scatter produced in the patient.
D. Increase film contrast.
E. Increase film blackening.

Answers overleaf

15A
TRUE—Field size is the most important factor in the production of scatter radiation. Reference *B*, p. 74.

15B
TRUE—The use of a compression band is the only way to obtain a reduction in part thickness. Reference *B*, p. 74.

15C
TRUE—Reference *B*, p. 101.

15D
TRUE—However, such a filter tends to remove primary and scattered radiation indiscriminately. Reference *A*, p. 250.

15E
FALSE—Because the radiation it removes would not have sufficient energy to reach the film. Reference *A*, p. 250.

16A
FALSE—More energetic radiation is produced which has a shorter wavelength. Reference *B*, p. 28.

16B
TRUE—Because more scatter will occur in a forward direction and be more likely to reach the film. Reference *A*, p. 68.

16C
FALSE—The amount of scatter decreases as the photon energy is increased. Reference *A*, p. 66.

16D
FALSE—Because scatter has no pattern and affects all areas of the film equally, it tends to decrease film contrast. Reference *A*, p. 244.

16E
TRUE—Because film blackening depends on the product of radiation intensity and exposure time. The radiation intensity varies as the square of the kVp. Reference *Y*, p. 10.

17 Concerning the half-value layer:

A. It is the thickness of a material required to reduce a narrow beam of X-rays to a half its original intensity.
B. It is a measure of radiation quality.
C. 10 half-value layers will reduce the intensity of a beam by a factor of about 1000.
D. It decreases for a polyenergetic beam with attenuation.
E. A beam can be attenuated to nothing by a thick layer of lead.

18 Concerning filtration:

A. Insulating oil is responsible for most inherent filtration.
B. In a compound filter of copper and aluminium, the copper is placed nearer the patient.
C. 0.5 mm of aluminium is suitable added filtration for tubes operating in the 70–100 kVp range.
D. It reduces the radiation dose to the skin.
E. It may necessitate a longer exposure.

Answers overleaf

17A
TRUE—Reference *A*, p. 61.

17B
TRUE—Reference *A*, p. 151.

17C
TRUE—The reduction in intensity is equal to 1/2 to the power of 10 i.e. 1024. Reference *A*, p. 63.

17D
FALSE—It increases because the beam becomes more energetic. Reference *B*, p. 410.

17E
FALSE—Because the reduction in intensity is exponential, an X-ray beam cannot be reduced to nothing. Reference *A*, p. 61.

18A
FALSE—The glass envelope is responsible for most inherent filtration. Reference *B*, p. 77.

18B
FALSE—The copper emits characteristic radiation of 8 keV which the aluminium then absorbs. Reference *B*, p. 78.

18C
FALSE—1.5 mm is suitable. Reference *B*, p. 79.

18D
TRUE—Reference *B*, p. 79.

18E
TRUE—Particularly when the kVp is low. Reference *B*, p. 80.

19 In the filtration of X-rays:

A. Tissue contrast is increased.
B. The photoelectric effect predominates.
C. A beryllium window results in less attenuation of the beam than one of glass.
D. A backing filter is required for 2 mm of aluminium.
E. 1.5 mm of aluminium is the recommended added tube filtration for an undercouch fluoroscopy tube.

20 In an unfocused grid:

A. The grid ratio is the distance between the strips divided by their width.
B. Lead strips 0.2 mm thick are commonly used.
C. More scatter radiation is removed by higher ratio grids.
D. The X-ray tube can be angled at 90 degrees to the direction of the lead strips.
E. The contrast improvement factor depends on the kVp at which it is measured.

Answers overleaf

19A
FALSE—There is a decrease in contrast because the mean kV of the beam is increased. However, this is significant only when the kVp is low. Reference *B*, p. 77.

19B
TRUE—Because the low kV radiation is principally absorbed. Reference *B*, p. 78.

19C
TRUE—Beryllium, with an atomic number of 4 and a k-absorption edge of 0.11 kV, hardly attenuates the beam at all. Reference *B*, p. 78.

19D
FALSE—No such filter is required because the characteristic radiation emitted by aluminium, being of low energy (1.5 kV), is absorbed in air. Reference *A*, p. 147.

19E
FALSE—2.5–4 mm of aluminium is recommended. This relatively large filtration is necessary in view of the short focus to object distance. Reference *H*, p. 28.

20A
FALSE—It is the ratio of the height of the strips to the distance between them. Reference *B*, p. 88.

20B
FALSE—The strips are about 0.05 mm thick. Reference *B*, p. 88.

20C
TRUE—Reference *B*, p. 88.

20D
FALSE—But it can be angled along the length of the grid strips. If it is angled at 90 degrees, then grid 'cut-off' occurs. Reference *B*, p. 89.

20E
TRUE—The contrast improvement factor is the ratio of the contrast with a grid to the contrast without a grid. It depends on the kVp, the field size and the phantom thickness. To permit comparison between grids, it is usually measured at 100 kVp. Reference *B*, p. 93.

21 The X-ray dose to the skin for a radiological examination is:

A. 0.8–1.2 rads during a chest radiograph.
B. Up to three times higher for a mass miniature chest film than for conventional radiography.
C. 1 rad for a minute of fluoroscopy during a barium meal.
D. Less when a high-ratio grid is used compared with a low-ratio grid.
E. Less if the area of the beam is reduced during fluoroscopy.

22 Concerning the effects of radiation:

A. High-speed electrons are less likely to produce ionization than slow-moving ones.
B. A high-speed electron produces more ionization at the beginning of its track.
C. The Bragg curve is the plot of relative ionization against distance travelled in a vacuum.
D. Fluorescence is normally produced by electrons falling directly from the conduction to the filled band.
E. The electron traps are normally empty in a phosphorescent material.

Answers overleaf

21A
FALSE—It is in the region of 0.2 rads. Reference *Z*1.

21B
TRUE—About 0.6 rads. Reference *Z*1.

21C
FALSE—The dose is about 4.5 rads per minute. Reference *Z*1.

21D
FALSE—Patient exposure is increased with an increase in ratio. This means that grid selection is a compromise between the improvement in image quality and the increase in exposure and skin dose. Reference *B*, p. 90.

21E
TRUE—It is important to keep the area of the beam and the screening time to a minimum.

22A
TRUE—Reference *A*, p. 82.

22B
FALSE—It will produce more ionization at the end of its track when it is moving slowly. Reference *A*, p. 82.

22C
FALSE—It plots distance travelled in air. Reference *A*, p. 83.

22D
FALSE—It is produced by electrons filling holes in the filled band from traps in the forbidden zone. Reference *A*, p. 90.

22E
TRUE—In contrast to a fluorescent material in which they are normally filled. Reference *A*, p. 92.

23 In the measurement of radiation:

A. The wall of a thimble chamber has a Z identical with that of air.
B. An exposure rate-meter requires a resistor in parallel to a voltmeter.
C. An exposure meter has the wall of an ionization chamber connected to one plate of a condenser.
D. Ionization chamber response increases with increasing wall thickness above a minimum set by the range of movement of the electrons.
E. A lead cylinder cathode increases the efficiency of a Geiger–Müller tube in the detection of gamma rays.

24 The thermoluminescent dosometer:

A. Employs a heat filter to reduce the dark current.
B. Demonstrates a linear relationship between absorbed dose and light emitted.
C. Has a scintillation crystal in front of the photocathode.
D. Demonstrates progressive glow curve fading after 24 hours.
E. Has the advantage over a film badge in that it can measure a very large exposure.

Answers overleaf

23A
FALSE—It is slightly lower than air (Z of air is 7.62 and that of the wall is 6). This is compensated for by the central electrode having a greater Z than air. Reference *A*, p. 107.

23B
TRUE—Whereas, an exposure meter has a condenser in parallel to the voltmeter. Reference *A*, p. 108.

23C
FALSE—The central electrode of the chamber is connected to the condenser. Reference *A*, p. 108.

23D
FALSE—Above a certain minimal thickness, the measured response decreases because of attenuation of the beam by the wall. Reference *A*, p. 114.

23E
TRUE—From 1 to 5%. Reference *A*, p. 119.

24A
TRUE—This allows for the passage of visible light, but not infra-red radiation which would cause a large dark current. Reference *A*, p. 126.

24B
FALSE—More light is produced per rad at higher doses, i.e. the relationship is supralinear. Reference *A*, p. 125.

24C
FALSE—The light from the thermoluminescent crystals is measured directly by the photocathode. Reference *A*, p. 125.

24D
FALSE—'Fading' takes place largely within 24 hours, after which the crystals are stable for many years. Reference *A*, p. 127.

24E
TRUE—Although designed to measure small doses. Reference *A*, p. 129.

25 Concerning X-ray film:

A. Supercoating consists of a thin layer of polyester.
B. Thiosulphate is the cause of the sensitivity specks in the silver halide lattice.
C. Speed is the reciprocal of the exposure required to produce a density of one above base and fog densities.
D. Exposing it to bright light after fixation will destroy the image contained by it.
E. Fog reduces the gradient of the characteristic curve mostly at low densities.

26 With X-ray film:

A. The gamma is the maximum slope of the characteristic curve.
B. Contrast is the difference in density between two points on the film.
C. The light-sensitive material in the emulsion is mostly silver iodide.
D. A fast film has smaller crystals in its emulsion than a slow film.
E. Double-coating of the emulsion doubles film contrast.

27 Concerning the characteristic curve of X-ray film:

A. An increase in the temperature of the developer increases the average gradient.
B. An increase in the temperature of the developer decreases base fog.
C. A film with an average gradient of one decreases subject contrast.
D. A film may have a high contrast and a wide latitude.
E. Contamination of the developer by fixer increases fog.

Answers overleaf

25A
FALSE—It is usually a layer of gelatin. Reference *B*, p. 129.

25B
FALSE—They are due to allylthiourea. Reference *B*, p. 127.

25C
TRUE—Reference *B*, p. 142.

25D
FALSE—But, of course, this would be true before fixation. Reference *A*, p. 168.

25E
TRUE—Reference *B*, p. 166.

26A
TRUE—The concept of average gradient is more useful, however. Reference *B*, p. 139.

26B
TRUE—Reference *B*, p. 139.

26C
FALSE—It is mostly silver bromide. About 1–10% is iodide. Reference *B*, p. 126.

26D
FALSE—Large crystals are more sensitive and confer greater speed on the film. Reference *A*, p. 183.

26E
TRUE—Film speed is also increased. Reference *A*, p. 190.

27A
TRUE—Reference *B*, p. 142.

27B
FALSE—It increases base fog. Reference *B*, p. 142.

27C
FALSE—It does not change subject contrast. A film with a gradient of less than one decreases subject contrast. Reference *B*, p. 140.

27D
FALSE—Film latitude and contrast are inversely related to each other. Reference *B*, p. 146.

27E
TRUE—Reference *B*, p. 166.

28 In the processing of X-ray film:

A. Development involves the oxidation of a silver ion.
B. Phenidone is used as a preservative.
C. Developers function at a pH range of 6–8.
D. Crystals that do not contain a latent image are not developed.
E. Retained fixing agent from poor washing will turn the film brown.

29 In silver recovery using high current density electrolysis:

A. Part of the fixer solution can be recycled.
B. The optimum pH is 7.5.
C. There is no simple means of estimating the silver content of fixer solution.
D. 98.5% of available silver can be recovered from waste fixer.
E. A stationary cathode is commonly used.

Answers overleaf

28A
FALSE—The developer donates an electron to the silver ion so that it becomes metallic silver. The silver is said to be 'reduced'. Reference *A*, p. 171.

28B
FALSE—This is one of the commonly used developers. Sodium sulphite acts as a preservative by combining with the oxidized developers and rendering them colourless. Reference *B*, p. 130.

28C
FALSE—The range is 10–11.5. Reference *B*, p. 130.

28D
FALSE—However, the reaction occurs at a much slower rate. Time is an important factor in development. Reference *B*, p. 130.

28E
TRUE—The retained thiosulphate will react with the silver to form brown silver sulphide. Reference *B*, p. 133.

29A
TRUE—Once its silver content has been reduced to $1\,g\,l^{-1}$, part of the fixer can be passed to a fixer recycle unit. Reference *Y*, p. 187.

29B
FALSE—It is 4.25. If it rises, then sulphiding may occur. The addition of acetic acid is used to keep the pH near the optimum. Reference *Y*, p. 187.

29C
FALSE—Test papers are used to estimate the silver content before and after electrolysis. Reference *Y*, p. 185.

29D
TRUE—Reference *B*, p. 184.

29E
FALSE—A rotating cathode is used to ensure that there is agitation of the fixer solution and that a constant supply of silver ions is brought into the vicinity of the cathode. Reference *B*, p. 186.

30 The metallic replacement method of silver recovery:

A. Can be used in conjunction with an automatic processor.
B. Requires electric power.
C. Uses steel wool.
D. Allows for recycling of fixer.
E. Can recover silver from the developer solution.

31 Intensifying screens:

A. Increase film speed.
B. Improve definition when compared with film exposed directly to X-rays.
C. Have an increased modulation transfer function with magnification.
D. Increase film contrast.
E. Are associated with greater cross-over of light when they have blue-emitting phosphors.

Answers overleaf

30A
TRUE—Reference *Y*, p. 185.

30B
FALSE—Reference *Y*, p. 185.

30C
TRUE—Reference *Y*, p. 187.

30D
FALSE—It is disposed of. Reference *Y*, p. 188.

30E
FALSE

31A
TRUE—Speed is defined as the reciprocal of the exposure required to produce a density of 1.0 above base and fog densities. Intensifying screens reduce the exposure necessary to achieve a density of 1 and, therefore, increase film speed. Reference *B*, p. 142.

31B
FALSE—Screens are a cause of image unsharpness because of light diffusion in the phosphor layer. Reference *B*, p. 172.

31C
TRUE—Because the screen deals with a lower image frequency when there is magnification. Reference *B*, p. 284.

31D
TRUE—Because they diminish the effect of scatter when compared with no-screen film. Reference *B*, p. 142.

31E
FALSE—Cross-over exposure is greater for the green-emitting phosphors. Reference *B*, p. 148.

32 In intensifying screens:

A. A phosphorescent material is used.
B. A reflecting coat of silver oxide is used.
C. Rare earth phosphors absorb a higher fraction of the incident X-ray beam than calcium tungstate.
D. Dye is used to minimize the effect of quantum mottle.
E. Dye is used to improve the sharpness of the image.

33 The use of rare-earth screens leads to:

A. Lower tube loading.
B. The use of smaller focal spots.
C. Less movement blur.
D. Less geometric unsharpness.
E. Reduction in quantum mottle.

Answers overleaf

32A

FALSE—The inorganic salts used in intensifying screens fluoresce, i.e. they are characterized by instantaneous light emission. Phosphorescent substances emit light for a longer time (greater than 10^{-8} seconds). Reference *B*, p. 107.

32B

FALSE—The reflecting coat is made of a white substance such as titanium oxide. Reference *B*, p. 108.

32C

TRUE—As a result of the favourable K absorption edges of the rare earth elements e.g. La, which has a k-binding energy of 38.9 keV and Gd, which has a k-binding energy of 50.2 keV. Reference *B*, p. 115.

32D

FALSE—Although, by absorbing a proportion of the emitted light, the use of a dye will necessitate a greater exposure. This will lead to a reduction in quantum mottle. Reference *B*, p. 112.

32E

TRUE—Light-absorbing dyes help to prevent diffusion of light in the phosphor layer. This acts to reduce the area of the film that can be exposed to light from any given point in the layer, and, therefore, the dye reduces screen unsharpness. Reference *B*, p. 112.

33A

TRUE—Because they reduce the exposures needed to produce a satisfactory radiograph. Reference *B*, p. 122.

33B

TRUE—Because smaller exposures are required.

33C

TRUE—Because exposure times can be reduced. Reference *B*, p. 122.

33D

TRUE—Because of the use of finer focuses.

33E

FALSE—The fast systems obtained with the new phosphors can lead to problems with noise. Reference *B*, p. 121.

34 Film sensitive to the blue region of the light spectrum should be used with:

A. Calcium tungstate screens.
B. Silver-activated zinc sulphide screens.
C. Zinc cadmium sulphide screens.
D. Barium strontium sulphate screens.
E. Terbium-activated screens.

35 The effects of quantum mottle are decreased:

A. By increasing the kVp when film is exposed using intensifying screens.
B. When image contrast is high.
C. For larger objects.
D. By widening the display window of a digital image.
E. By the use of frame integration (the averaging of several frames) in digital subtraction.

Answers overleaf

34A
TRUE—Mean emission occurs at 430 nm, which is in the blue region. Reference *B*, p. 109.

34B
TRUE—This screen phosphor is used in photofluorography. Reference *B*, p. 122.

34C
FALSE—This is the phosphor used in the output screen of image intensifiers; it emits in the yellow–green region. Reference *B*, p. 122.

34D
TRUE—The peak for the spectral emission of this phosphor is at 380 nm. Reference *B*, p. 118.

34E
FALSE—This is the activator for rare-earth screens and emits at 544 nm, which is in the yellow–green region. Reference *B*, p. 117.

35A
FALSE—Because the higher kVp X-rays produce a higher screen intensification factor and reduce the number of photons of X-radiation used to make the exposure. Reference *B*, p. 168.

35B
TRUE—High-contrast images are sharpness limited. The effects of quantum mottle are greater for low-contrast images. Reference *B*, p. 436.

35C
TRUE—Because an object with a large area has a greater inherent subject contrast and is less likely to be mimicked by quantum mottle. Reference *B*, p. 439.

35D
FALSE—A narrow window increases the image contrast. This has the effect of decreasing the effects of quantum mottle. A wide window produces the opposite situation. Reference *B*, p. 436.

35E
TRUE—All types of noise are reduced by this method. Reference *B*, p. 440.

36 In the physics of vision:

A. The retinal rods have the highest minimum threshold to light.
B. Acuity is greatest for photopic vision.
C. The eye is able to store information for up to 2 seconds.
D. Rods are relatively insensitive to red light.
E. Peripheral vision is sharper for faint shadows on a screen.

Answers overleaf

36A

FALSE—Cones have the highest threshold to light. Reference *A*, p. 341.

36B

TRUE—Photopic vision, which is due to the presence of cones in the retina, occurs with the levels of brightness seen in daytime. Acuity is greater for this, which explains the need to increase the brightness levels in fluoroscopy to that required for cone vision. Reference *A*, p. 352.

36C

FALSE—The time over which the eye is able to store information is referred to as the integration time. This is only 0.2 seconds. Hence, gazing for a prolonged period at a poorly illuminated fluoroscopic image does not supply additional information to the eye. Reference *B*, p. 187.

36D

TRUE—So that the dark-adapting radiologist could wear red goggles. Reference *A*, p. 345.

36E

TRUE—Because the concentration of rods is greater in the periphery of the retina and they are more sensitive to low levels of illumination. Reference *A*, p. 348.

37 In an image intensifier:

A. The output screen is coated with a thin layer of aluminium.
B. X-rays are focused on to the output phosphor.
C. The anode has a positive potential of 250 V.
D. The small size of the output phosphor compared with that of the input screen produces a gain in brightness.
E. Cesium iodide has a higher photon-to-light conversion factor than zinc cadmium sulphide.

38 Circular tomography, when compared to linear tomography, provides:

A. More uniformity of blurring of objects outside the focal plane.
B. Less distinct blur margins.
C. Greater expense.
D. Thinner tomographic sections.
E. Shorter exposure times.

Answers overleaf

37A

TRUE—On the side of the photocathode. It prevents light produced in the output phosphor from passing retrogressively to the photocathode. Reference *B*, p. 192.

37B

FALSE—Electrons are guided on to the output phosphor by the electrostatic focusing lens. Reference *B*, p. 190.

37C

FALSE—The potential is 25 000 V (25 kV). Reference *B*, p. 192.

37D

TRUE—This is known as minification gain and is equal to the square of:

$\frac{d_i}{d_O}$ where d_i is the diameter of the input screen and d_O the diameter of the output screen. Reference *B*, p. 193.

37E

FALSE—The advantages of cesium iodide are the improved quantum detection, the better resolution and the better contrast. The improved quantum detection reflects the more favourable k-absorption edges and the greater packing density. Reference *B*, p. 205.

38A

TRUE—Parasite lines do not occur in circular tomography. Reference *B*, p. 250.

38B

FALSE—The blur margins are more distinct. Reference *B*, p. 251.

38C

TRUE—Reference *B*, p. 251.

38D

FALSE—The section thickness depends on the arc of tube swing and not on the shape of tube movement. Reference *B*, p. 247.

38E

FALSE—The longer exposure times which are required in circular tomography and other complex movements are a drawback. This is because they increase the risk of movement blur. Reference *B*, p. 251.

39 In tomography:

A. Objects outside the focal plane are equally blurred.
B. An angle of swing of 10 degrees gives a section 12 mm thick.
C. An angle of swing of 20 degrees gives a section 3.4 mm thick.
D. Multifilm cassettes improve contrast.
E. Multifilm cassettes reduce the radiation dose to the patient per film exposed.

40 In the technique of subtraction:

A. The gamma of the film used to form the mask is one.
B. The mask cannot be processed in an automatic processor.
C. Subtraction film has emulsion on both sides.
D. A second-order image is obtained by superimposing the first mask and the scout film and exposing them to a white-light source.
E. Opaque foreign bodies can be located in the eye.

Answers overleaf

39A
FALSE—The degree of blurring depends upon the distance from the focal plane and the distance from the film. Reference *B*, p. 246.

39B
FALSE—It gives a section 6.9 mm thick. Reference *B*, p. 248 (Fig. 18-9).

39C
TRUE—Although the section is not much thinner than that obtained with a 10 degree angle, the blurring of objects outside the focal plane is significantly greater. Reference *B*, p. 248 (Fig. 18-9).

39D
FALSE—Their major disadvantage is that there is uncontrolled scatter radiation which diminishes film quality. Reference *B*, p. 257.

39E
TRUE—Although the dose per exposure is increased so as to penetrate the layers, the dose per film is decreased. Reference *B*, p. 256.

40A
TRUE—So as to cause no exaggeration or lessening of densities on the scout film. Reference *B*, p. 292.

40B
FALSE—This is no longer true. Reference *B*, p. 292.

40C
FALSE—The emulsion is single sided. Reference *B*, p. 293.

40D
TRUE—A higher degree of subtraction is obtained, but there is an increase in image unsharpness. Reference *Y*, p. 257.

40E
TRUE—The position of gaze is changed between the scout film and a second film. Any opaque foreign bodies will not then be subtracted. Reference *B*, p. 293.

41 The 'ten-day rule':

- **A.** Should be applied to radiography of the paranasal sinuses.
- **B.** States that the referring clinician is responsible for ascertaining the date of the LMP.
- **C.** Should be applied to females who have been taking the contraceptive pill for 3 months and found it effective.
- **D.** Should be applied to females who have had an IUCD inserted 1 month previously.
- **E.** Should be applied to females who are menstruating at the time of the examination.

42 In xeroradiography:

- **A.** A light-tight cassette is required.
- **B.** There is a narrow exposure latitude.
- **C.** A low initial photoreceptor plate voltage gives increased contrast.
- **D.** Corona discharge is used at several stages in the formation of a xeroradiograph.
- **E.** A greater radiation dose is seen during mammography than with film–screen combinations.

Answers overleaf

41A

FALSE—The rule is applied to plain radiography of the abdomen and pelvis and to special examinations, such as barium enemas, which involve radiation to structures in those areas. Reference: The Royal College of Radiologists: Recommendations on the implementation of 'The Ten-Day Rule'. *British Journal of Radiology*; **49**: 201–2 (1976).

41B

TRUE—Reference: *British Journal of Radiology*; **49**: 201–2 (1976).

41C

FALSE—Reference: *British Journal of Radiology*; **49**: 201–2 (1976).

41D

TRUE—The 10 day rule is not applicable to those who have had an IUCD for over 3 months. Reference: *British Journal of Radiology*; **49**: 201–2 (1976).

41E

FALSE—Reference: *British Journal of Radiology*; **49**: 201–2 (1976).

42A

TRUE—Light will discharge the ions from the surface of the selenium. Reference *B*, p. 300.

42B

FALSE—There is a wide exposure latitude. Reference *B*, p. 316.

42C

FALSE—Low initial voltage gives low contrast, and vice versa. Reference *B*, p. 313.

42D

TRUE—Corona discharge is the ionization of air and the outward movement of the charged particles around a wire to which a large potential has been applied. It is used to charge the plate; in the pre-transfer and transfer stages when the developed plate and paper are brought together so that the image can be recorded; and in the final cleaning of the plate. Reference *B*, p. 305 and 317.

42E

TRUE—Reference *B*, p. 319.

43 In xeroradiography:

A. Crystalline selenium is used.
B. The sulphur impurities in the selenium play a role in image formation.
C. The selenium layer is 400 μm thick.
D. Edge enhancement of the image is seen.
E. A high back-bias voltage applied to the aluminium backing during development increases contrast.

44 In CT:

A. A CT number is proportional to the linear attenuation coefficient.
B. A CT number is accurate to 5 units for a magnifying constant of 2000.
C. Third-generation scanners do not have linear-type movements.
D. The size of a single picture element is known as the matrix size.
E. Patient exposure is increased when increasing voxel size for constant counting statistics.

Answers overleaf

43A
FALSE—Amorphous selenium is used because it has the properties of a photoconductor, i.e. it is a substance that conducts after exposure to radiation. Crystalline selenium, which is the most stable form, is a conductor of electricity. Reference *B*, p. 303.

43B
FALSE—The selenium must be pure because the presence of any impurity increases the dark decay rate. Reference *B*, p. 303.

43C
FALSE—Selenium shows maximal sensitivity to X-rays in the energy range employed in diagnostic radiology when it has a thickness of 130 μm. This thickness is therefore used. Reference *B*, p. 304.

43D
TRUE—This occurs because toner is attracted away from the low-voltage side to the high-voltage side of any boundary where there is an abrupt change in charge density. Reference *B*, p. 312.

43E
FALSE—It decreases contrast. Reference *B*, p. 313.

44A
TRUE—Reference *B*, p. 338.

44B
FALSE—It is accurate to within 0.5%, which is equal to 10 units for a magnifying constant of 2000. Reference *B*, p. 338.

44C
TRUE—In contrast to first- and second-generation scanners which do. Reference *B*, p. 325.

44D
FALSE—The term matrix size refers to the number of points in a picture matrix, e.g. the size is 6400 for a 80 × 80 matrix. Reference *B*, p. 343.

44E
FALSE—The exposure is increased when maintaining the counting statistics in a smaller voxel. Reference *B*, p. 342.

45 In the original EMI CT scanner:

A. A pixel was a 3 × 3 × 13 mm block of tissue.
B. Voxel size could be altered once the transmission data had been collected by the computer.
C. A 120 kVp beam was used.
D. Sodium iodide scintillation crystals were used.
E. A fan-shaped beam was used.

46 Radioactivity:

A. Is more likely to occur when a sample of ^{60}Co is heated.
B. Is a random process.
C. Occurs when a positron and electron annihilate each other.
D. Falls exponentially for a given sample of a radionuclide.
E. Is associated with a range in water of 2 cm for beta particles.

Answers overleaf

45A

FALSE—These figures represent the size of a volume element (voxel) scanned in the patient. The picture element produced by the computer, and representing a cross-section of 3 × 3 mm, is a pixel. Reference *B*, p. 323.

45B

FALSE—The size of a volume element is determined by the width of the X-ray beam. Once data have been collected, their representation is open to alteration by the computer. Reference *B*, p. 324.

45C

TRUE—Reference *B*, p. 324.

45D

TRUE—The alternative is to use gas-filled ionization chambers. Reference *B*, p. 324.

45E

FALSE—This was a feature of later scanners. The first scanners had a sharply collimated, pencil-like X-ray beam. Reference *B*, p. 324.

46A

FALSE—Radioactivity concerns the interactions within an unstable nucleus, and occurs in isolation to external influences. Reference *C*, p. 7.

46B

TRUE—Reference *C*, p. 8.

46C

FALSE—Electromagnetic radiation is emitted. Reference *C*, p. 10.

46D

TRUE—Reference *A*, p. 29.

46E

FALSE—The approximate range, which is dependent on energy, is 0.43 cm. Reference *A*, p. 27 (Table III).

47 Comparing the radionuclides $^{99}Tc^{m}$ and $^{113}In^{m}$:

A. $^{113}In^{m}$ has the longer half-life.
B. $^{99}Tc^{m}$ emits the lower-energy gamma radiation.
C. $^{99}Tc^{m}$ loses less of its radiation in internal conversion.
D. $^{99}Tc^{m}$ is preferred because its parent ^{99}Mo has the longer half-life.
E. Only $^{113}In^{m}$ gives rise to a stable daughter.

48 In the use of radionuclides:

A. A $^{99}Tc^{m}$ generator has ^{99}Mo absorbed on to aluminium oxide.
B. Generators must be protected from light.
C. Saline is used to elute an indium generato..
D. A fine collimator improves the resolution of a scanner.
E. Beta-rays contribute little to measured activity.

Answers overleaf

47A

FALSE—It has a half-life of 100 minutes, whereas that of $^{99}Tc^{m}$ is 6 hours. Reference *C*, p. 19.

47B

TRUE—140 keV as against 392 keV. Reference *C*, p. 19.

47C

TRUE—Reference *C*, p. 19.

47D

FALSE—^{99}Mo has a half-life of 2 days and 19 hours, whereas ^{113}Sn has a much longer half-life of 118 days. This longer half-life favours the use of indium because it means that a generator need be purchased every 4 months or so, rather than once a week or so for technetium. Reference *C*, p. 19.

47E

TRUE—The product of the decay of $^{99}Tc^{m}$ is slightly active. Reference *C*, p. 19.

48A

TRUE—Reference *C*, p. 18.

48B

FALSE—However, they must be sterile if the eluent is to be used for an intravenous injection.

48C

FALSE—Dilute hydrochloric acid is used. It is important that the correct eluent be used, because otherwise the parent may be eluted in significant amounts. Reference *C*, p. 20.

48D

TRUE—The collimator attempts to reduce the radiation reaching the scanner from areas distant to the region of interest. Reference *A*, p. 406.

48E

TRUE—This is because they rarely penetrate as much as 1 cm. However, they contribute considerably to the radiation dose received by the patient. Reference *C*, p. 12.

49 Concerning the isotopes of iodine:

A. ^{132}I has a half-life of 2.26 hours.
B. ^{125}I is a beta emitter.
C. ^{123}I emits gamma radiation with an energy of 159 keV.
D. ^{123}I has a half-life of 13 days.
E. They must be administered intravenously.

50 In the Geiger–Müller tube:

A. The central wire is the cathode.
B. Gas-amplification occurs.
C. The anode and cathode are contained in a vacuum.
D. Sensitivity is greater to high-energy radiation.
E. The long 'dead-time' results in too low a reading.

Answers overleaf

49A
TRUE—Reference *C*, p. 185.

49B
FALSE—It emits gamma radiation of low energy (37 keV). Reference *D*, p. 42.

49C
TRUE—Reference *D*, p. 42.

49D
FALSE—The half-life is 13 hours. This isotope is preferred for thyroid scanning. Reference *D*, p. 42.

49E
FALSE—They are given by mouth. Reference *C*, p. 185.

50A
FALSE—It is the anode. Reference *A*, p. 118.

50B
TRUE—Reference *A*, p. 118.

50C
FALSE—They are enclosed within a thin glass envelope which contains an inert gas. Reference *A*, p. 118.

50D
FALSE—Because high-energy radiation tends to pass through the tube without detection. Reference *A*, p. 119.

50E
TRUE—The dead-time is normally about 300 μs. Reference *A*, p. 119.

51 In the Geiger–Müller tube:

A. Alcohol vapour is added.
B. Counting is performed with the voltage in the plateau region.
C. The gas is at low pressure.
D. The potential difference is 25 kV.
E. The energy of the radiation can be measured.

52 In a photomultiplier tube:

A. Electrons are accelerated through a series of dynodes.
B. External light is not excluded.
C. The sides of the phosphor are whitened to form a reflective layer.
D. Radiation of different energies can be distinguished apart.
E. The dead-time is the same as that in a Geiger–Müller tube.

Answers overleaf

51A
TRUE—Or halogen gas. Reference *A*, p. 118.

51B
TRUE—The count-rate is independent of voltage in this region. Reference *A*, p. 118.

51C
TRUE—Reference *A*, p. 118.

51D
FALSE—The potential difference is 200–400 V for halogen-filled tubes, and 900–1500 V for alcohol-filled tubes. Reference *A*, p. 118.

51E
FALSE—Which is one of the reasons why the tube has been superseded for radioactivity measurements. Reference *A*, p. 119.

52A
TRUE—Reference *A*, p. 120.

52B
FALSE—Light coming from outside the tube which is incident on the photocathode will produce a pulse. It is excluded by a thick metal housing and a thin layer of opaque material over the face of the phosphor. Reference *A*, p. 120.

52C
TRUE—To reflect back any light that might otherwise have escaped. Reference *B*, p. 329.

52D
TRUE—Because the size of the electrical pulse depends on the amount of light reaching the photocathode. This in turn depends on the amount of energy absorbed from the incident photon. Reference *B*, p. 121.

52E
FALSE—It is shorter. This is an advantage over the Geiger–Müller tube. Reference *B*, p. 121.

53 In a gamma camera:

A. There is a light guide between the crystal and the photomultiplier tube.
B. Collimators are unnecessary.
C. Resolution is increased by increasing the number of photomultiplier tubes.
D. The scintillation crystal consists of sodium iodide.
E. Some light from a scintillation is received by every photomultiplier tube.

54 Comparing a gamma camera with a rectilinear scanner:

A. The camera is less efficient at detecting low-energy radiation (less than 70 keV).
B. The camera is more easily coupled to an on-line data processor.
C. The scanner is better for dynamic studies.
D. Patient positioning is easier with the scanner.
E. Field uniformity is greater with the camera.

Answers overleaf

53A
TRUE—Reference *A*, p. 411.

53B
FALSE—The use of collimators is intended to match, as far as possible, the pattern of scintillations in the crystal with the distribution of radioactivity in the patient. Reference *A*, p. 412.

53C
TRUE—Reference *A*, p. 415.

53D
TRUE—Reference *A*, p. 411.

53E
TRUE—The amount received by each varies in inverse proportion to the square of the distance from the scintillation. Reference *A*, p. 413.

54A
TRUE—Reference *C*, p. 46.

54B
TRUE—Reference *C*, p. 46.

54C
FALSE—It cannot be used for this. Reference *C*, p. 46.

54D
FALSE—Reference *C*, p. 46.

54E
FALSE—It is equal at best to that seen with a scanner. Reference *C*, p. 46.

55 In a vidicon camera:

A. The tube is surrounded by two pairs of electric coils.
B. A graphite plate forms the dot picture.
C. The cathode-coil assembly forms an electron gun.
D. The electron beam hits the target at an angle of 60 degrees.
E. The anode is a solid metal cylinder.

56 Concerning diagnostic ultrasound:

A. Modern piezoelectric crystals are quartz compounds.
B. A piezoelectric crystal with a high Q factor makes a good receiver of echoes.
C. The diameter of the crystal determines its resonant frequency.
D. Increasing the frequency increases the absorption of the sound.
E. The absorption coefficient for fat is higher than that for lung.

Answers overleaf

55A
TRUE—These are focusing and deflecting coils. Reference *B*, p. 230.

55B
FALSE—It forms the signal plate which gives the video signal. The dot picture forms on the target, which is made of a film of a photoconductive material (e.g. antimony trisulphate) suspended as globules in a mica matrix. Reference *B*, p. 231.

55C
TRUE—Reference *B*, p. 231.

55D
FALSE—The anode straightens out the beam so that its angle of incidence is 90 degrees. Reference *B*, p. 231.

55E
FALSE—It is a wire mesh. Reference *B*, p. 231.

56A
FALSE—Lead zirconate titanate is used. Reference *B*, p. 357.

56B
FALSE—The Q factor refers to the length of time that a crystal 'rings'. An undamped element with a high Q will produce a long pulse of sound in response to an electrical stimulus. It will be unavailable to receive returning echoes during this time. Reference *B*, p. 360.

56C
FALSE—The thickness of the crystal determines the resonant frequency. Reference *B*, p. 358.

56D
TRUE—Absorption and frequency are directly related. Reference *B*, p. 369.

56E
FALSE—At a frequency of 1 MHz, the coefficient for fat and lung are 0.63 and 41 dB cm^{-1} respectively. Reference *B*, p. 369.

57 Concerning the physics of sound:

A. The human ear can hear sound frequencies in the 20 000–50 000 Hz range.
B. The bel is an absolute measure of sound-beam energy.
C. A piezoelectric crystal heated to the Curie temperature loses its properties.
D. The thickness of a piezoelectric crystal is half the wavelength of the sound it produces.
E. The wavelength in soft tissue of sound generated by a 1.5 MHz transducer is 3 mm.

58 The velocity of sound in human soft tissue:

A. Is 1450 $m\,s^{-1}$.
B. Is the same as that in water.
C. Is proportional to frequency in the diagnostic ultrasound range.
D. Is less than that in the skull.
E. Is inversely related to the compressibility of the medium.

Answers overleaf

57A
FALSE—The range of hearing in the human is from about 16 to 20 000 Hz. Ultrasound has a frequency greater than the upper limit of hearing, by definition. Medical ultrasound is in the 1–20 MHz range. Reference *B*, p. 353.

57B
FALSE—It is a relative measure of the power of two sound beams expressed as a logarithm of base 10. Reference *B*, p. 355.

57C
TRUE—Reference *B*, p. 358.

57D
TRUE—The thickness will be less than 1 mm for transducers producing sound frequencies greater than 2 MHz. Reference *B*, p. 359.

57E
FALSE—It is 1 mm. This is calculated from the equation $c = \lambda\nu$, where c = velocity ($\mathrm{m\,s^{-1}}$); λ = wavelength (m); and ν = frequency (Hz).

For soft tissue: $1540 = 1.5 \times 10^6\lambda$,

$\therefore \lambda = 1.0 \times 10^{-3}\mathrm{m}$.

Reference *B*, p. 354.

58A
FALSE—It is 1540 $\mathrm{m\,s^{-1}}$. 1450 $\mathrm{m\,s^{-1}}$ is the velocity in fat. Reference *B*, p. 353.

58B
TRUE—Reference *B*, p. 353.

58C
FALSE—It is independent of frequency and is a function of the physical properties of the medium through which the sound is passing. Reference *B*, p. 353.

58D
TRUE—The velocity in the skull is 4080 $\mathrm{m\,s^{-1}}$. Reference *B*, p. 353.

58E
TRUE—Reference *B*, p. 354.

59 In ultrasound:

A. Sound waves are transmitted through a liquid as transverse waves.
B. Reflection is proportional to the acoustic impedance mismatch at a tissue interface.
C. About 80% of the beam is reflected back from a muscle–bone interface.
D. Acoustic impedance increases with increasing density if the sound velocity is constant.
E. Acoustic impedance is the reciprocal of the absorption coefficient for a given medium.

60 In diagnostic ultrasound:

A. Side-to-side (lateral) resolution is improved by increasing the crystal diameter.
B. The diameter of the crystal determines the length of the near (Fresnel) zone.
C. Depth (axial) resolution is determined by the length of the sonic pulse.
D. The angle of dispersion in the far zone increases with increased crystal diameter.
E. The angle of dispersion in the far zone increases with increase in wavelength.

Answers overleaf

59A

FALSE—The waves are longitudinal in type. This means that the motion of the particles is parallel to the direction of the wave. Reference *B*, p. 352.

59B

TRUE—It also varies with angle of incidence. Reference *B*, p. 365.

59C

FALSE—About 40% is reflected. This can be calculated from the acoustic impedance values for the two media (Z_1 and Z_2) and the equation

$$R = \left[\frac{(Z_2 - Z_1)}{(Z_2 + Z_1)}\right]^2$$

where R = percentage of the beam reflected. Reference *B*, p. 366.

59D

TRUE—The impedance is the product of density and the velocity of sound in a medium. Reference *B*, p. 365.

59E

FALSE—Reference *B*, p. 365.

60A

FALSE—To resolve objects in the horizontal plane, the beam must be narrower than the space separating them. Reference *B*, p. 381.

60B

TRUE—A narrow transducer, while it has high lateral resolution, is not able to penetrate usefully to deep-lying structures. Reference *B*, p. 362.

60C

TRUE—The spatial pulse length depends on the wavelength and the number of waves in the pulse. Reference *B*, p. 378.

60D

FALSE—The angle is inversely related to the crystal diameter. Reference *B*, p. 364.

60E

TRUE—The equation determining the angle of dispersion is:

$$\text{Sine of angle} = 1.22\,\frac{\lambda}{D}$$

where λ = wavelength; and D = diameter of transducer. Reference *B*, p. 364.

61 In the display of an ultrasound image:

A. A-mode utilizes a moving time base.
B. B-mode produces an image of a section or slice through the patient.
C. Returning echoes can be displayed either as white or black dots.
D. A digital scan converter uses a binary code storage.
E. The time gain compensation graph is linear.

62 The Doppler shift for a 10 MHz transducer:

A. Is a frequency change.
B. Falls within the hearing range of the human ear.
C. Is greatest when the beam is perpendicular to the reflecting surface.
D. Is inversely proportional to the velocity of blood flow at a given angle.
E. Is detected by the use of two piezoelectric elements.

Answers overleaf

61A
FALSE—This is seen in TM mode. Reference *B*, p. 372.

61B
TRUE—Reference *B*, p. 379.

61C
TRUE

61D
TRUE—Reference *B*, p. 374.

61E
FALSE—Although commonly represented as a straight line, the curve of the time gain compensator is exponential. Reference *B*, p. 375.

62A
TRUE—Reference *B*, p. 385.

62B
TRUE—Reference *B*, p. 386.

62C
FALSE—It is greatest when there is an acute angle of reflection. This is opposite to the situation in abdominal ultrasound. Reference *B*, p. 386.

62D
FALSE—It is directly proportional. Reference *B*, p. 386.

62E
TRUE—Two are used. There is overlap of the beam regions. Reference *B*, p. 386.

63 In grey-scale, real-time ultrasound:

A. Returning echoes are assigned a shade of grey according to their intensity.
B. At least 16 frames per second are needed for a flicker-free display.
C. Image resolution improves when frame frequency is increased.
D. An increase in the number of lines per field of view requires a decrease in the frame frequency.
E. Decreasing the angle of a sector scan has no effect on image resolution.

64 In mechanical sector scanning using a single oscillating unenclosed transducer crystal:

A. A plastic focusing lens is used.
B. Frame rate is independent of rate of oscillation.
C. No vibrations are felt by the patient.
D. A trapezoid image is produced.
E. A mirror system can be used to direct the sound beam.

Answers overleaf

63A
TRUE—This is a definition of grey-scale ultrasound. Reference *B*, p. 374.

63B
TRUE—Reference *B*, p. 390.

63C
FALSE—A fast frame rate is needed when fast moving structures, such as the heart, are imaged. Reference *B*, p. 391.

63D
TRUE—This inverse relationship exists because time is needed for a sound pulse to leave a transducer and then return to it from a structure. As resolution improves when the number of lines is increased, a compromise has to be reached when imaging a fast-moving structure. Reference *B*, p. 391.

63E
FALSE—It improves resolution by increasing the line frequency. The field of view is decreased. Reference *B*, p. 391.

64A
FALSE—This is used in a linear array scanner. Reference *B*, p. 394.

64B
FALSE—It depends on oscillation rate. Reference *B*, p. 392.

64C
FALSE—No vibrations are felt from the sector scanners which employ an oil or water to enclose the crystal. Reference *B*, p. 392.

64D
FALSE—A sector image is produced. A trapezoid image is seen with the enclosed crystal scanner because the sound beam has to traverse the enclosing oil. Reference *B*, p. 392.

64E
TRUE—Reference *B*, p.392.

65 An electronic focus in a linear array scanner:

A. Improves resolution.
B. Stimulates the inner elements of the transducer a few nanoseconds before the outer elements to produce a focused beam.
C. Cannot vary the depth of focus.
D. Is used in liver scans with a transducer frequency of about 2–3.5 MHz.
E. Can be manipulated to give a sector scan.

66 Concerning the effects of ultrasound:

A. Heat results from the interaction of ultrasound and tissue.
B. 'Cavitation' occurs in the lung.
C. The intensity of the sound is unrelated to the chance of biological effects.
D. Medical ultrasound is safe.
E. It does not cause ionization.

Answers overleaf

65A
TRUE—In the plane parallel to the image plane. Azimuthal resolution is said to be improved. Reference *B*, p. 395.

65B
FALSE—The outer elements are the first to be stimulated. Reference *B*, p. 395.

65C
FALSE—The depth of focus, which is the range of distances over which the image is sharp, can be varied electronically. Reference *B*, p. 395.

65D
TRUE—Reference *B*, p. 395.

65E
TRUE—But the technology is costly. This type of scanning is known as steered or phase array. Reference *B*, p. 396.

66A
TRUE—The amount of heat increases with increasing power of the beam. Reference *T*, p. 29.

66B
FALSE—This is the formation of microbubbles in liquids and is seen with high-intensity sound at low frequency, i.e. not the type used in medical diagnosis. Reference *T*, p. 29.

66C
FALSE—The evidence available suggests that there is a threshold at a peak intensity of 100 m cm^{-2} below which no detectable effects are likely. Reference *T*, p. 30.

66D
TRUE—Reference *T*, p. 30.

66E
TRUE

67 According to the Code of Practice, the lead gloves and body aprons used in diagnostic radiology:

A. Must provide adequate protection from the unattenuated primary beam.
B. Must have a lead equivalent of 0.15 mm or more.
C. Should be examined radiographically at least annually.
D. Are required to have a minimum lead equivalent equal to the minimum required for the apron on the fluoroscopy table.
E. Should be worn by a parent supporting a child during radiography.

68 Concerning measurements:

A. The becquerel is the rate of disintegration of 1 gram of uranium 235.
B. A becquerel is 1×10^3 disintegrations per second.
C. A roentgen is equivalent to 100 J kg^{-1}.
D. The dose equivalent is obtained by multiplying the absorbed dose by the quality factor of the radiation.
E. The radiation dose limit for the gonads in the occupationally exposed is 5 rems per annum.

Answers overleaf

67A
FALSE—They are designed to protect against primary radiation transmitted through the patient and from scatter. Reference *Z*, section 3.16, p. 23.

67B
FALSE—The minimum lead equivalent is 0.25 mm. Reference *Z*, section 3.16, p. 23.

67C
TRUE—To ensure that their function has not been impaired by cracks in the material. Reference *Z*, section 3.16, p. 23.

67D
FALSE—The apron at the fluoroscopy table must have 0.5 mm of lead or more. Reference *Z*, section 3.12, p. 21.

67E
TRUE—Child patients should be held by a parent or guardian. If possible, a radiographer should not support a child patient. Reference *Z*, section 3.3, p. 15.

68A
FALSE—The previously accepted unit, the curie, was based on the disintegration of 1 g of radium. Reference *A*, p. 43.

68B
FALSE—It is one disintegration per second. Reference *A*, p. 43.

68C
FALSE—The roentgen is the unit of exposure. It is equal to 2.58×10^{-4} coulomb per kg of air. The rad, which is a unit of absorbed dose, is the dose of any type of ionizing radiation accompanied by the absorption of 100 ergs of energy per gram. The rad is to be superseded by the gray, which is equal to 1 J kg^{-1} and 100 rads. Reference *A*, p. 99.

68D
TRUE—The rem and the sievert are the units of dose equivalent. Reference *B*, p. 403.

68E
TRUE—Reference *Z*, p. 79 (Table B1).

69 In radiation protection:

A. The quality factor for X-rays is five.
B. The quality factor of radiation is directly related to linear energy transfer.
C. The maximum accumulated whole-body dose permissible for a worker aged 38 years is 100 rem (1 Sv).
D. The annual whole body dose limit for the general population is one-fifth that for the occupationally exposed.
E. The hands of the occupationally exposed may receive up to 75 rems (0.75 Sv) in 1 year.

70 An individual's exposure to natural background radiation:

A. Contributes the same to the genetically significant dose as occupational sources.
B. Arises partly from ^{40}K in ingested food and water.
C. Is highest at sea level.
D. Has an average value which is estimated to be 1.25 rem.
E. Is smaller than that from man-made sources (e.g. atomic fall-out).

Answers overleaf

69A
FALSE—It is one. Reference *Z*, p. 81.

69B
TRUE—the linear energy transfer is the amount of energy deposited in tissue per unit length. Reference *B*, p. 403.

69C
TRUE—Based on the dose limit of 5 rem (0.05 Sv) each year after the age of 18. Reference *B*, p. 405.

69D
FALSE—The annual limit is 0.5 rem (0.005 Sv), or one-tenth that for the occupationally exposed. Reference *B*, p. 406.

69E
TRUE—Reference *B*, p. 406 (Table 26–5).

70A
FALSE—Natural radiation accounts for about 100 times the dose received from occupational exposure. This is because the number of people receiving an occupational dose (e.g. radiologists) up to the maximum permitted (5 rem) is small. Therefore, the genetically significant dose is much smaller than that from the natural environment. Reference *B*, p. 404.

70B
TRUE—An internal dose arises from radionuclides in food, water and air. These are chiefly radium and thorium and their decay products ^{40}K and ^{14}C. Reference *B*, p. 404.

70C
FALSE—It is higher at altitude. Reference *B*, p. 404.

70D
FALSE—125 mrem is the estimated value. Reference *B*, p. 404.

70E
FALSE—The man-made sources of radiation account for about 4 mrem exposure. Reference *B*, p. 404.

71 When setting up radiographic apparatus for digital subtraction angiography:

A. It is essential to have a generator capable of giving repeatable exposures.
B. Specially designed X-ray tubes are needed.
C. Very small focal spots are essential.
D. A high-quality image intensifier is needed.
E. The advantage of having a plumbicon television camera is its high lag.

72 Nuclear spin (I):

A. Is directly proportional to the maximum detectable nuclear angular momentum.
B. Is equal and opposite to electron spin for all atoms.
C. Is a whole number if the mass number is odd.
D. May have a value of 3.6.
E. Causes precession in a magnetic field.

Answers overleaf

71A
TRUE—Otherwise contrast differences on the films will be different and subtraction will not work properly. Reference *B*, p. 421.

71B
FALSE—Standard tubes already used in angiography are suitable. Reference *B*, p. 421.

71C
FALSE—Because focal spot size is not a limiting factor to resolution. A very small focal spot is actually undesirable because of the reduced tube-loading characteristics. Reference *B*, p. 421.

71D
TRUE—Reference *B*, p. 422.

71E
FALSE—It has low lag. This means that there is less motion blurring when the camera is moved rapidly during fluoroscopy. However, it is easier to detect quantum mottle with a plumbicon camera. Reference *B*, p. 422.

72A
TRUE—Reference *B*, p. 464.

72B
FALSE—Electron spin is always a half whereas nuclear spin is either zero, a multiple of a half, or a whole number. Reference *B*, p. 464.

72C
FALSE—It is a multiple of a half in this situation. Reference *B*, p. 464.

72D
FALSE—The number is always zero or divisible by a half. Reference *B*, p. 464.

72E
TRUE—Reference *B*, p. 465.

73 Magnetic dipole moment:

A. Is measured in joules per tesla.
B. Is given in Bohr magnetons for electrons.
C. Is the same for neutrons and protons.
D. Is directed at 90 degrees to the spin axis of a spinning particle.
E. May be zero for a nucleus.

74 In a given magnetic field, the Larmor frequency of a nucleus:

A. Is the frequency of precession.
B. Depends on the gyromagnetic ratio.
C. Is constant for elements in the same periodic group.
D. Is greater than the frequency of radiation absorbed in a spin transition.
E. Is in the radiofrequency range for a hydrogen atom if the field strength is 1.0 tesla.

Answers overleaf

73A
TRUE—Reference *B*, p. 467.

73B
TRUE—Reference *B*, p. 467.

73C
FALSE—Reference *B*, p. 467.

73D
FALSE—It is in the same direction. Reference *B*, p. 467.

73E
TRUE—Such an atom will be undetectable by NMR. Reference *B*, p. 468.

74A
TRUE—A nucleus that has a nuclear spin will also have a magnetic dipole moment. It will become aligned, therefore, in an externally applied magnetic field, such that the angular moment will be at right angles to the axis of the magnetic field. The motion of the spinning nucleus about this axis is called precession. The frequency of precession is the Larmor frequency. Reference *B*, p. 470.

74B
TRUE—According to the equation:

$$\nu_L = \gamma \frac{H}{2\pi}$$

where ν_L = Larmor frequency; H = magnetic field; γ = gyromagnetic ratio. Reference *B*, p. 470.

74C
FALSE—It is unique for any nucleus. Reference *B*, p. 471.

74D
FALSE—It is exactly equal. Reference *B*, p. 473.

74E
TRUE—It is 42 MHz. Reference *B*, p. 473.

75 After excitation of a substance by a 90 degrees radiofrequency magnetic pulse:

A. The signal produced by the free return of the magnetization to the pre-excitation state is free induction decay.
B. T_2 represents the gradient of a straight line.
C. T_2 is known as the spin–spin relaxation time.
D. T_2 may be larger than T_1.
E. The difference between T_2 and T_1 tends to be greater in solids.

76 The resistive coil air core magnet:

A. Consumes current for a fraction of the time that a magnetic field is produced.
B. Produces field strengths of 3–4 tesla.
C. Uses liquid helium and nitrogen for cooling.
D. Can achieve a greater field uniformity than superconducting magnets.
E. Has an improved signal-to-noise ratio when magnetic field strength is increased.

Answers overleaf

75A
TRUE—Reference *B*, p. 480.

75B
FALSE—It represents the time constant of an exponential function as the in-phase dipoles become randomized. Reference *B*, p. 480.

75C
TRUE—It is the decay constant perpendicular to the applied external magnetic field. Reference *B*, p. 480.

75D
FALSE—It cannot be. Reference *B*, p. 482.

75E
TRUE—Reference *B*, p. 482.

76A
FALSE—Current is consumed for the whole time. Reference *B*, p. 490.

76B
FALSE—They produce fields of 1–2 tesla. Reference *B*, p. 490.

76C
FALSE—This applies to superconducting magnets. Reference *B*, p. 491.

76D
FALSE—The superconducting magnets achieve more field uniformity. Reference: James, A. E., *et al.* Nuclear magnetic resonance imaging: the current state. *Am. J. Roent*; **138**:201–10 (1981).

76E
TRUE—Reference *B*, p. 488.

77 In NMR imaging:

A. Gradient magnetic fields are used to provide spatial resolution.
B. Increased speed of image acquisition is seen compared with CT.
C. Cortical bone gives a strong signal.
D. Cross-sectional images in any orientation are possible.
E. Different pulse sequences are used to reduce the biological hazard.

78 When X-ray film is stored:

A. Low humidity tends to increase film fog.
B. Non-screen film suitable for automatic processing has a short half-life.
C. The background radiation should ideally be 5 mR per hour or less.
D. The maximum temperature should be 21°C.
E. It should be handled at the edges.

Answers overleaf

77A
TRUE—Gradient magnetic fields permit interrogation of a point, a line or a plane. The thickness of a plane in which dipoles find the resonance condition is determined by the gradient of the field. Reference *B*, p. 497.

77B
FALSE—It may take 1–2 minutes to collect data from a plane about 2 mm thick. The longer the time, the better the image quality. Reference *B*, p. 499.

77C
FALSE—There is no signal because of the low mobile proton population (only about 12%).

77D
TRUE

77E
FALSE—There is no proven biological hazard. Possible effects detrimental to health might arise from:

1. The strength of the constant magnetic field.
2. The radiofrequency irradiation.
3. The time-varying magnetic field.

Reference *B*, p. 500.

78A
FALSE—High humidity increases base fog. Reference *Y*, p. 48.

78B
TRUE—Because the emulsion has been sensitized to compensate for the decrease in the coating weight of silver halide. Reference *Y*, p. 39.

78C
FALSE—It should ideally be less than 5 μR per hour. Reference *Y*, p. 51.

78D
TRUE—Reference *Y*, p. 50.

78E
TRUE—And stored on edge. Reference *Y*, p. 43.

79 In the construction and operation of a darkroom:

A. A lead lining to the cassette hatch door is usually unnecessary.
B. Barium plaster may be needed on the walls.
C. Orthochromatic film must be handled in complete darkness.
D. 6 m^2 floor space is adequate.
E. An actinic marker can be recessed in the working surface.

80 The Wisconsin cassette:

A. Measures tube mA.
B. Contains an intensifying screen.
C. Uses a single emulsion film.
D. Has a lead mask in which a series of holes have been drilled.
E. Uses a series of copper step-wedges.

Answers overleaf

79A
FALSE—As the cassette hatch usually opens into a radiography room, it is desirable to have lead lining to the door so as to reduce the radiation exposure inside the darkroom. Reference *Y*, p. 173.

79B
TRUE—To reduce the radiation levels within the room. Reference *Y*, p. 51.

79C
FALSE—A safelight at the red end of the spectrum can be used. Panchromatic film has to be handled in the dark. Reference *B*, p. 148.

79D
FALSE—9 m^2 is the minimum acceptable floor space. The ceiling should be 3 m high. Reference *Y*, p. 170.

79E
TRUE—An actinic marker is a device for identifying film with the patient's name. It exposes a small area of the film to light. Reference *Y*, p. 172.

80A
FALSE—It measures kVp. Reference *Y*, p. 290.

80B
TRUE—The screen is covered by five optical attenuators which give a series of reference densities on the exposed film. Reference *Y*, p. 290.

80C
FALSE—Standard, duplitized screen-type film is used. Reference *Y*, p. 290.

80D
TRUE—Reference *Y*, p. 290.

80E
TRUE—The densities on the film achieved through the copper are compared directly with the reference density resulting from film exposure through the optical attenuators. Reference *Y*, p. 291.

III. RADIOLOGICAL TECHNIQUES AND RADIOGRAPHY

2 Severe reactions to urographic contrast media:

A. Cause more deaths in patients over 50 years of age.
B. Occur in 90% of injections where there is a history of a previous reaction.
C. May produce a prolonged nephrogram.
D. Are invariably preceded by a rash or vomiting.
E. Are an indication for the use of intravenous chlorpheniramine.

Answers overleaf

2A
TRUE—Severe reactions are defined as those where there is fear for the patient's life. They appear to be more frequent in the older age groups and have been shown to cause more deaths in people over 50 years of age. Reference *U*, p. 6.

2B
FALSE—The risk of recurrence appears to be about 35%. Reference *U*, p. 18.

2C
TRUE—A persistently dense nephrogram and poor pelvicaliceal opacification will be found if the patient is profoundly hypotensive, which may occur as part of a severe reaction to contrast. Reference *S*, p. 223.

2D
FALSE—Although severe reactions may be presaged by nausea, vomiting or a skin rash, this is not invariable. Reference *U*, p. 8.

2E
FALSE—Antihistamines may be of value in the treatment of urticaria, e.g. chlorpheniramine maleate 10 mg intravenously. They are of no value either in the prophylaxis or treatment of severe reactions. Reference *S*, pp. 222–3.

3 Concerning reactions to urographic contrast media:

A. Bronchospasm is more likely with a sodium than with a meglumine salt.
B. They may occur when only 1 ml has been injected.
C. Rigors are seen in patients given large doses.
D. A perivenous injection will invariably be detected by the swelling it causes at the injection site.
E. They may be delayed in onset.

4 Sodium iothalamate:

A. Does not cross the normal blood–brain barrier.
B. Is isomeric with sodium diatrizoate.
C. Is preferred to meglumine iothalamate in arthrography.
D. Causes haemolysis.
E. Is suitable for myelography.

Answers overleaf

3A
FALSE—The incidence of bronchospasm is four times greater with meglumine media. Reference *U*, p. 19.

3B
TRUE—The use of such small amounts as a 'test injection' serves no useful function because it may itself cause a severe reaction or even death. Conversely, a severe reaction may occur with a large injection following an uneventful test dose. Reference *U*, p. 29.

3C
TRUE—And more commonly with meglumine salts. They may rarely occur after a small injection. Reference *U*, p. 11.

3D
FALSE—A perivenous injection may not be clinically apparent. It may cause severe, persistent arm pain. This pain is most severe when the contrast medium has a high sodium content, e.g Conray 420. Reference *U*, p. 12.

3E
TRUE—Although reactions usually occur during or a few minutes after the injection, they may rarely be delayed in onset. Reference *U*, p. 6.

4A
FALSE—The normal blood–brain barrier is deficient at a number of sites. This is the central fact in Lalli's theory that reactions to contrast agents are mediated via the nervous system. Reference: Contrast media reactions: data analysis and hypothesis. *Radiology*; **134**:1–12 (1980).

4B
TRUE—Reference *S*, p. 339.

4C
FALSE—The sodium salt may cause severe pain if extra-articular injections occur.Reference *K*, p. 57.

4D
TRUE—Reference *S*, p. 340.

4E
FALSE—A non-ionic contrast agent is indicated. Reference *S*, p. 265.

5 The sodium salt of diatrizoic acid:

A. Is more viscous than the meglumine salt.
B. Causes less of a diuresis than the meglumine salt.
C. May rarely cause a peripheral neuropathy.
D. May rarely cause salivary gland enlargement.
E. Is predominantly bound to plasma protein.

6 In intravenous urography:

A. Contrast is freely filtered at the glomerulus.
B. Water deprivation results in a denser nephrogram.
C. A rapid injection of a dose of contrast gives a denser nephrogram than a slower one.
D. A standard dose of contrast supplies 40 g of iodine in a 70 kg man.
E. The kidneys in infants are better demonstrated when the stomach is distended with air.

Answers overleaf

5A
FALSE—The meglumine salt is more viscous. Reference *E*, p. 599 (Table 29.1).

5B
TRUE—Which is the reason why sodium salts are preferred for urography. Reference *S*, p. 217.

5C
FALSE

5D
TRUE—This usually occurs 2–4 days after the injection. Reference *U*, p. 15.

5E
FALSE—Less than 1% is plasma-protein bound. Reference: Lasser, E. C., *et al.* The significance of protein binding of contrast media in Roentgen diagnosis. *Am. J. Roent*; **87**:338–60 (1962).

6A
TRUE—Reference *S*, p. 216.

6B
FALSE—The 'tubular' nephrogram seen after an intravenous injection of contrast is the result of that freely filtered contrast in the renal tubules. It is independent of the degree of hydration. Reference *S*, p. 217.

6C
TRUE—The concentration of contrast in the glomerular filtrate, and the density of the nephrogram, depends on the peak plasma concentration and the renal blood flow. The former will depend upon the dose and rate of injection. Reference *S*, p. 216.

6D
FALSE—The standard dose is 300 mg iodine per kg, which is 21 g in a man of 70 kg. Reference *S*, p. 217.

6E
TRUE—This supplies a 'window' through which the kidneys are seen. This can be achieved in infants who are being bottle fed by feeding them in the supine position immediately before and after the injection. More air is swallowed by tilting the bottle the wrong way. In older children, a carbonated drink or air introduced down a nasogastric tube can be used. Films should be taken AP and oblique (left side raised). This latter is more likely to project the gastric 'window' over the right kidney. Reference *J*, p. 43.

7 In intravenous urography:

A. Iohexol causes an electrocardiographic change less often than sodium iothalamate.
B. Prone films are of no value.
C. Elevating the arm helps to alleviate pain extending proximally from the injection site.
D. Opacification of the gut occurs if there is renal failure.
E. Precipitation of renal failure in diabetics is a known risk of the procedure.

8 An empty bladder is required before:

A. Lymphography.
B. Pelvic ultrasound.
C. Intravenous urography.
D. CT of the pelvis.
E. Hysterosalpingography.

Answers overleaf

7A

TRUE—Iohexol was shown to cause very few ECG changes. Reference: Heron, C. W., Underwood, S. R. and Dawson, P. Electrocardiographic changes during intravenous urography: a study with sodium iothalamate and iohexol. *Clinical Radiology*; **35**:137–41 (1984).

7B

FALSE—They are often useful for demonstrating the ureters. Reference *S*, p. 220.

7C

TRUE—This phenomenon, which results from stasis of contrast, is more likely to occur with sodium salts of high concentration, e.g. Conray 420. Reference *S*, p. 222.

7D

TRUE—Hepatic excretion of the contrast occurs. Reference *E*, p. 826.

7E

TRUE—It is best to avoid urography in diabetics with renal impairment. Reference *S*, p. 215.

8A

TRUE—Because the procedure may take a long time to complete, it is best to have the patient empty their bladder at the beginning. Reference *S*, p. 184.

8B

FALSE—A full bladder is essential in pelvic ultrasound. If the bladder is empty, small bowel will fill the space and cause difficulties. Furthermore, the full bladder acts as an acoustic window. Reference *F*, p. 23.

8C

TRUE—Urine will dilute the contrast and prevent good mucosal coating on the after-micturition film. Reference *S*, p. 216.

8D

FALSE—As with pelvic ultrasound, the distended bladder displaces small bowel out of the pelvis and facilitates identification of other structures. Reference *Q*, p. 393.

8E

TRUE—Because a full bladder displaces the uterus and interferes with its delineation by contrast. Reference *J*, p. 85.

9 In retrograde urography in an undistended system:

A. Ureteric perforation may occur.
B. Acute renal failure is a complication of the procedure.
C. Contrast with 300 mg iodine per 100 ml is used.
D. Filling of the pelvicaliceal system is best performed with a head-down tilt.
E. 50 ml of contrast is usually needed to fill the pelvicaliceal system adequately.

10 In urethrography of the male:

A. The Knutsson clamp should be used when there is a phimosis.
B. A viscous contrast medium gives good distension of the urethra.
C. The bulbo-urethral glands are usually demonstrated.
D. The verumontanum is seen in the normal patient.
E. The procedure should be stopped if intravasation occurs.

Answers overleaf

9A
TRUE—This is more likely with a rigid catheter. Reference *S*, p. 227.

9B
TRUE—Rarely. Reference *S*, p. 227.

9C
FALSE—A contrast medium with a low concentration of iodine, such as Urografin 150, is used so that non-opaque calculi are not obscured. Reference *S*, p. 227.

9D
TRUE—Reference *S*, p. 225.

9E
FALSE—5–10 ml is adequate. The injection should not be fast or made with more than minimal pressure. Reference *S*, p. 227.

10A
FALSE—The clamp cannot be used in this situation, because the correct application of the clamp demands retraction of the prepuce. A Foley catheter with its balloon lying in the navicular fossa is indicated for this problem. Reference *S*, p. 241.

10B
TRUE—Which is a major advantage over simple water-soluble contrast. Reference *S*, p. 242.

10C
FALSE

10D
TRUE—This is a longitudinal ridge in the prostatic urethra.

10E
TRUE—Recent instrumentation predisposes to this complication. Bleeding may accompany it. Reference *S*, p. 243.

11 Gastrografin is preferred to barium in the examination of the alimentary tract:

A. In neonates.
B. In cases of suspected oesophagobronchial fistula.
C. In perforation of the stomach or duodenum.
D. When demonstrating oesophageal varices.
E. When looking for an anastomotic leak in the colon.

12 In a double-contrast barium meal:

A. A low mA and high kVp should be used ideally.
B. The visualization of the areae gastricae indicates good coating.
C. A phototimer should be positioned over the barium pool.
D. Rugal folds on the posterior stomach wall appear as radiolucent defects in the supine position.
E. Transverse folds are not seen in the normal oesophagus.

Answers overleaf

11A
FALSE—The high osmolality of the conventional water-soluble contrast media causes problems when used in the very young because of the fluid they draw into the gut lumen (Reference *S*, p. 19). There may be a place for the low osmolal contrast media in the investigation of the neonatal gut. Reference: Ratcliffe, J. F. The use of ioxoglate in the paediatric gastrointestinal tract: a report of 25 cases. *Clinical Radiology*; **34**:579–83 (1983).

11B
FALSE—It should not be used where there is a risk of it entering the bronchial tree and of causing pulmonary oedema. Reference *S*, p. 19.

11C
TRUE—When plain films fail to show free gas. Reference *S*, p. 19.

11D
FALSE—The oesophagus should be in a relaxed state with a good coating of barium. Reference *S*, p. 15.

11E
TRUE—Reference *S*, p. 47.

12A
FALSE—The mA should be set as high as possible so as to reduce the exposure time and risk of movement blur. A low kVp is desirable to achieve maximum contrast. Reference *I*, p. 20.

12B
TRUE—When there is good coating, the mucosal surface has a uniform greyness, and the mamillated surface of the stomach mucosa (the areae gastricae) can be seen. Reference *I*, p. 14.

12C
FALSE—As it is the areas seen in double contrast that interest us, it is important to position the phototimer over such areas and not over the barium pool. Otherwise the film will be over-exposed. Reference *N*, 20.4, p. 672.

12D
TRUE—They form a linear defect in the barium puddle. Folds on the anterior wall form two thin white lines. The differing appearances permit separation of posterior and anterior wall lesions. Reference *I*, p. 23.

12E
FALSE—Delicate transverse folds are occasionally seen. They are usually mid-oesophageal in location and are believed to represent the contractions of the muscularis mucosae. Reference *I*, p. 81.

13 In a barium meal:

A. The supine RAO/LPO position is used to show the lesser curve '*en face*'.
B. A prominent longitudinal fold is present in the second part of the duodenum.
C. Filling of the cap with barium occurs more reliably with glucagon than with hyoscine *N*-butyl bromide.
D. The oesophagus is seen in double contrast if barium is drunk whilst holding the nose.
E. Glucagon is considerably cheaper than hyoscine *N*-butyl bromide.

14 In the barium infusion technique of examining the small bowel:

A. Patient preparation is unnecessary.
B. A Malström–Westerman tube is used.
C. Passage of the tube through the pyloric sphincter is best performed with the patient lying on his right side.
D. A hydrometer is used to check that the relative density (specific gravity) of the barium suspension is 1.25–1.32.
E. A rate of infusion of 75 ml per minute to a total volume of 1200 ml is suitable.

Answers overleaf

13A
FALSE—The antrum is shown in double contrast by this position. The LAO/RPO position demonstrates the lesser curve *en face*. Reference *I*, p. 70 (Fig. 3-1I).

13B
TRUE—In 90% of individuals. Reference *I*, p. 339.

13C
FALSE—The opposite is true because one of the effects of Buscopan is relaxation of the pylorus. Reference *S*, p. 15.

13D
TRUE—Because the patient has to swallow air. Reference *S*, p. 15.

13E
FALSE—The opposite is true.

14A
FALSE—The patient should be fasted overnight. Reference *S*, p. 22.

14B
FALSE—A Bilbao–Dotter tube or modification is used. Reference *S*, p. 23.

14C
FALSE—It is better to have the patient lying on his left side. This is because the gastric antrum and duodenal cap fill with air in this position and facilitate the passage of the tube through the sphincter. Reference *S*, p. 23.

14D
TRUE—The relative density is considered important. Reference *S*, p. 27.

14E
TRUE—Reference *S*, p. 27.

15 The transit of barium through the small bowel during a follow-through examination is accelerated by:

A. Intravenous metoclopramide.
B. Oral metoclopramide.
C. Food residue in the ileo-caecal region.
D. Barium that has been warmed to body temperature.
E. Hyoscine *N*-butyl bromide.

Answers overleaf

15A
TRUE—A significant difference has been shown in the stomach emptying time and in the transit time to the caecum. The trial was double-blind and placebo controlled. Reference: James, W. B. and Hume, R. Action of metoclopramide on gastric emptying and small bowel transit time. *Gut*; **9**: 203–5 (1968).

15B
TRUE—In a study of 110 patients, which was not placebo controlled, 20 mg given immediately prior to meal and follow-through led to barium reaching the caecum in 75 minutes in all but 12 patients. Reference: Kreel, L. The use of oral metoclopramide in the barium meal and follow-through examination. *British Journal of Radiology*; **43**:31–5 (1970).

15C
FALSE—This can delay transit considerably. A cathartic should be given prior to an examination of the small bowel. Reference *S*, p. 23.

15D
FALSE—The motility of the small bowel may be increased by the administration of cold isotonic saline. Reference *H*, p. 864.

15E
FALSE—An anticholinergic drug such as this will delay the transit of barium.

16 In adrenal venography:

A. The left adrenal vein is more difficult to catheterize than the right.
B. Venous sampling is an integral part of the procedure.
C. A loop is formed in the inferior vena cava when using a cobra end-hole catheter to cannulate the left adrenal vein.
D. Approximately 8 ml of contrast are required for the right adrenal vein.
E. A rapid injection is given to provoke hormone production.

17 Intraosseus phlebography:

A. Requires local anaesthesia.
B. Should be avoided in patients with unfused epiphyses.
C. Should be performed with the patient prone to improve demonstration of the internal iliac vein.
D. May cause a fat embolus.
E. Is complicated by bone infarction in 5–10% of cases.

Answers overleaf

16A
FALSE—The right is the harder to catheterize. This is because it originates from the inferior vena cava and has a variable site. Reference *K*, p. 50.

16B
TRUE—Adrenocortical hormone assays are important in the diagnosis of adrenal tumours. Reference *S*, p. 121.

16C
TRUE—The catheter is advanced along the left renal vein to its more peripheral tributaries. The loop is then formed in the vena cava by advancing the catheter against the resistance of its tip. The direction of the tip changes to point superiorly. Movements are then 'reversed', the tip of the catheter moving out of the renal vein when the catheter is advanced at the groin and vice versa. Reference *K*, p. 48.

16D
FALSE—2 ml is needed for the right and about 8 ml for the left. Reference *E*, p. 811.

16E
FALSE—The injection is given slowly after a test injection under fluoroscopic control. Rupture of the glands is a complication of rapid injection. Reference *K*, p. 47.

17A
FALSE—It is a painful technique that requires general anaesthesia. Reference *L*, p. 42.

17B
TRUE—Because inadvertent extravasation around the epiphysis may impair its subsequent growth. Reference *L*, p. 42.

17C
FALSE—This position gives a better display of the external and common iliac veins. The patient is placed supine to show the internal iliac vein fully. Reference *L*, p. 45.

17D
TRUE—In which case, the urine, blood and sputum should be examined for globules of fat. Reference *L*, p. 62.

17E
FALSE—Lea Thomas has not encountered a case in over 1000 examinations. Reference *L*, p. 62.

18 In angiography:

A. The axillary artery is more prone to spasm than the femoral artery.
B. The renal arteries are approached from the right axilla rather than the left.
C. Guide wires have a core of three inner wires.
D. Bonded heparin-coated catheters reduce the incidence of thrombus formation.
E. The puncture site for antegrade femoral studies is distal to that used for retrograde procedures.

19 The following are appropriate injections of contrast:

A. 50–100 ml ioxoglate 320 at 14 ml s^{-1} for bilateral lower limb arteriography.
B. 25 ml iopamidol 300 for selective renal arteriography.
C. 10 ml meglumine iothalamate 280 into a frontal vein for orbital venography.
D. 50 ml ioxoglate 320 at 20 ml s^{-1} for superior mesenteric arteriography.
E. 10 ml sodium iothalamate 420 for common carotid arteriography.

Answers overleaf

18A
TRUE—Therefore, catheter manipulation and time of the procedure should be kept to a minimum when using the axillary artery. The femoral route is chosen where possible. Reference *S*, p. 102.

18B
FALSE—The right side is used for the ascending aorta and selective studies in the head and neck. The left is used for the descending and abdominal aorta and its branches. Reference *S*, p. 103.

18C
FALSE—They have two inner wires and an outer circular wire which binds them tightly. One of the inner wires tapers and terminates a few centimetres from the tip which allows for flexibility. Reference *S*, p. 99.

18D
TRUE—But they are not easily pre-shaped. Guide wires similarly coated also reduce the incidence of thrombotic complications. Reference *S*, p. 125.

18E
FALSE—Because the needle is directed towards the feet, the puncture site for an antegrade study should be proximal to that used for conventional retrograde angiograms. If the site of puncture is too distal, the deep or superficial femoral arteries may be entered. Reference *K*, p. 125.

19A
TRUE—Reference *S*, p. 107 (Table 8.1).

19B
FALSE—A smaller quantity such as 12 ml is suitable. Reference *S*, p. 112 (Table 8.3).

19C
TRUE—Orbital venography has been largely superseded by computed tomography. Reference *S*, p. 299.

19D
FALSE—This is too rapid. A more appropriate rate would be 8 $ml\,s^{-1}$. Reference *S*, p. 112 (Table 8.3).

19E
FALSE—This would be unsuitable because of its sodium content and its high iodine concentration. Meglumine iothalamate 280 may be used, but the new low-osmolal contrast media are the preferred agents. Reference *S*, p. 286.

20 In translumbar aortography:

A. A systolic blood pressure greater than 200 mm Hg is a contra-indication to the procedure.
B. An aortic aneurysm may be safely punctured.
C. The low approach is often easier than the high approach in patients with severe atheroma.
D. A high puncture is made opposite the disc at L1/2.
E. Slight caudal angulation of the needle is employed.

21 In translumbar aortography:

A. A test injection of a test dose may be omitted if there is free back-flow of blood.
B. Damage to the spinal cord is a complication of the procedure.
C. Dissection is usually a minor complication.
D. A gradual advance of the needle once aortic pulsation is felt is important for the success of the puncture.
E. A sub-intimal injection of a test dose is usually painful.

Answers overleaf

20A
TRUE—Reference *K*, p. 17.

20B
FALSE—This would be dangerous and is contra-indicated. Reference *S*, p. 105.

20C
FALSE—The low approach is often more difficult because the inferior part of the lumbar aorta tends to be more variable in site and because its lumen tends to be narrower and more likely to be atheromatous. Reference *J*, p. 215.

20D
FALSE—The level of puncture is T12. The needle is introduced just below the 12th rib (about 2 cm) and 8–10 cm from the midline. Reference *K*, p. 18.

20E
FALSE—The needle is introduced at right angles or with a cranial angulation. The latter is usual when a high puncture is performed. Reference *S*, p. 105.

21A
FALSE—It is a crucial part of the procedure and the single most important factor in making it safe. It allows a check to be made that the needle has not entered a branch artery and that it is well positioned in the lumen. Reference *J*, p. 217.

21B
TRUE—Rarely. Reference *U*, p. 66.

21C
TRUE—Reference *U*, p. 64.

21D
FALSE—Once the pulsation can be felt, the operator should make short 2–3 mm stabbing thrusts. This will ensure puncture of one wall. If a gradual advance is made, then the nearer wall may be slowly compressed such that the needle will pass through both walls together. Reference *J*, p. 214.

21E
FALSE—It is usually painless. There will be a dense persistence of contrast at the end of the needle. Pain suggests that a periaortic injection has occurred, in which case the test film will show less-dense persistence of contrast spreading out into the soft tissues. Reference *J*, p. 217.

22 In cardiac angiography:

A. A J-guide may help catheter advancement where there is tortuosity of the iliac arteries.
B. Hypotension may occur during the procedure.
C. Dissection of a coronary artery is rarely of clinical importance.
D. Bradycardia does not usually require treatment.
E. 20 ml of contrast is a suitable injection for demonstrating the left coronary artery.

23 In cardiac angiography:

A. The Sones technique includes the use of a catheter exchange sheath in the femoral artery.
B. A pigtail catheter is safest for a left ventricular angiogram.
C. A cine-film frequency of 15 frames per second is usually adequate for examination of the coronary arteries.
D. Contrast injected into a coronary artery should rapidly disperse.
E. Perforation of an artery or cardiac chamber may occur.

Answers overleaf

22A

TRUE—Atherosclerotic disease predisposes to arterial dissection. A J-guide reduces this risk compared with a straight guide. The guide should be advanced gently and without the use of force when there is tactile recognition of a resistance to its progress. Reference *S*, p. 126.

22B

TRUE—There are a number of factors that may cause a fall in blood pressure. It should be recognized and, if possible, treated: it may precede cardiac arrest. Reference *U*, p. 91.

22C

FALSE—Urgent surgical intervention may be required (Reference *S*, p. 163). Dissection is an uncommon complication of coronary arteriography, but cardiac arrest usually ensues.

22D

FALSE—It should be treated, for it may herald asystole. Reference *U*, p. 91.

22E

FALSE—This is too large an amount. The quantity and speed of injection, usually 2–9 ml by hand, may be decided upon from the appearances of a test injection of 1–2 ml. Reference *S*, p. 160.

23A

FALSE—It uses a single catheter, introduced from a cut-down on the brachial artery, for catheterization of the left ventricle and coronary arteries. Reference *S*, p. 159.

23B

TRUE—Because of its flexibility and side holes, a pigtail catheter is less likely to recoil during an injection and become malpositioned in a small vessel or the wall of a cardiac chamber. Reference *S*, p. 148.

23C

FALSE—30–60 frames per second are required. Reference *B*, p. 223.

23D

TRUE—If it does not do so, then a partial occlusion of the coronary artery by the catheter may have occurred. The catheter should be withdrawn immediately. Reference *S*, p. 160.

23E

TRUE—This is more likely to occur with stiff and end-hole catheters. It may be recognized by a change in pressure or difficulty in withdrawing blood on aspiration. Reference *S*, p. 159.

24 In pulmonary angiography:

A. A pigtail catheter is placed midway between the pulmonary valve and bifurcation.
B. 30 ml of contrast is injected via a power injector over 3 seconds into the main artery.
C. AP and lateral films are required.
D. Balloon-occlusion catheters can be used to provide improved image quality.
E. Rupture of the right ventricular chordae tendinae can occur.

25 In inferior mesenteric angiography:

A. The artery arises from the left anterolateral aspect of the aorta.
B. The artery arises at L2.
C. A sidewinder catheter should not be used.
D. Films are taken with the patient in the RPO position.
E. 35 ml iopamidol at 14 ml s^{-1} is a suitable injection.

Answers overleaf

24A
TRUE—Reference *S*, p. 155.

24B
FALSE—45 ml in 1.5 seconds is an appropriate quantity and rate. Reference *S*, p. 155.

24C
FALSE—The lateral film is of no value because of superimposition. The AP view is sufficient, although an oblique view may be obtained if required. Reference *S*, p. 155.

24D
TRUE—They can be used in selected parts of the pulmonary arterial tree which are known to be abnormal from a previously performed perfusion scan. Reference: Bynum, L. J., *et al.* Radiographic techniques for balloon-occlusion pulmonary angiography. *Radiology*; **133**:518–20 (1982).

24E
TRUE—This occurs as the pigtail is withdrawn, and is avoided by using the guide to straighten out the end of the catheter. Reference *S*, p. 156.

25A
TRUE—Reference *S*, p. 118.

25B
FALSE—It arises at L3. Reference *S*, p. 118.

25C
FALSE—It is commonly used. Its shape can be formed in the arch of the aorta before catheterization of the artery, and it should be straightened before removal at the end of procedure.

25D
FALSE—The patient should be in the LPO position to open out the artery.

25E
FALSE—25 ml at 8 $ml s^{-1}$ is appropriate. Reference *S*, p. 112 (Table 8.3).

26 In percutaneous splenoportography (PSP):

A. The puncture is made in the anterior axillary line if the spleen is impalpable.
B. The inferior mesenteric vein is seen in the normal examination.
C. The left gastric vein is better demonstrated than by the venous phase of a coeliac angiogram in the normal patient.
D. The normal pulp pressure is less than 20 mm Hg.
E. Gelfoam is used to reduce bleeding.

27 Oral cholecystographic contrast media:

A. Differ from water-soluble contrast media in that the carbon-5 position in the benzene ring is unsubstituted.
B. Are lipid soluble.
C. Have peak concentrations in the bile ducts at 10–14 hours after administration.
D. Do not usually undergo a enterohepatic circulation.
E. Are removed from the blood by passive diffusion.

Answers overleaf

26A
FALSE—The smaller the spleen, the more posteriorly is the puncture made. When the spleen is impalpable, the puncture is made in the posterior axillary line with slight cephalad and anterior angulation to the needle. Reference *J*, p. 268.

26B
FALSE—Reference *H*, p. 918.

26C
FALSE—It is not normally seen at PSP. Reference *S*, p. 165.

26D
FALSE—It is normally less than 11 mm Hg. Reference *S*, p. 169.

26E
TRUE—And should be used routinely in patients at particular risk of bleeding. Reference *S*, p. 169.

27A
TRUE—This causes them to be bound to plasma protein, reducing their glomerular filtration and leading to their preferential excretion by the liver. Reference *S*, p. 60.

27B
TRUE—Iopanoic acid is the most lipid soluble of the oral cholecystographic media. Reference *S*, p. 60.

27C
FALSE—As far as ipodate is concerned, the peak concentration in the ducts occurs at about 3 hours. Maximum levels in the gall bladder occur at 14–19 hours depending on the particular contrast medium. Reference *S*, p. 62.

27D
FALSE—There is some deconjugation of the glucuronide and absorption in the ileum. Reference *S*, p. 62.

27E
FALSE—An active transport mechanism is used. It is rate limited. Reference *S*, p. 62.

28 In oral cholecystography:

A. The contrast agents are uricosuric.
B. Smoking may interfere with opacification of the biliary tree.
C. The prone oblique view demonstrates the bladder neck.
D. Screening is not helpful.
E. Renal excretion of contrast medium indicates hepatic disease.

29 In intravenous cholangiography:

A. Monomeric compounds are used.
B. Glucagon is contra-indicated.
C. Opacification of the biliary tree is unlikely when the serum bilirubin is over 68 $\mu mol\,l^{-1}$.
D. Contrast refluxing into the first part of the duodenum simulates an opacified gall bladder in post-cholecystectomy patients.
E. An erect film of the gall bladder is performed at 24 hours if there is stratification of bile on the first erect film.

Answers overleaf

28A
TRUE—This may account for the occasional nephrotoxicity of the contrast agents. A good fluid intake should be encouraged and does not interfere with the activity of the media. Reference: Mudge, G. H. Uricosuric action of cholecystographic agents. *New England Journal of Medicine*; **284**:929–33 (1971).

28B
TRUE—It is advisable to ask patients not to smoke prior to the examination. Reference *S*, p. 63.

28C
FALSE—It demonstrates the fundus. This, being the most anterior part of the gall bladder, is where the contrast collects in the prone position. The neck and body are best seen on the supine oblique (30 degrees left side raised) position. Reference *J*, p. 94.

28D
FALSE—Screening is the most effective way of obtaining films in which the gall bladder is not obscured by overlying bowel gas. Reference *J*, p. 94.

28E
FALSE—There is a variable rate of renal excretion in the normal patient, e.g. 21–57% of ipodate is removed by the kidneys. Reference *S*, p. 62.

29A
FALSE—The intravenous media have dimeric molecules with high aqueous solubility. Reference *S*, p. 69.

29B
FALSE—There appears to be improved visualization of the biliary tree after injection of glucagon. Reference *S*, p. 71.

29C
TRUE—Reference *S*, p. 71.

29D
TRUE—It may be misinterpreted as a gall bladder. Oral contrast will demonstrate the position of the duodenum in such cases. Reference *J*, p. 102.

29E
TRUE—The stratification or layering phenomenon is thought to be due to poor mixing of contrast laden new bile and old bile. Mixing will have occurred on the later film. Reference *S*, p. 73.

30 In the radiological investigation of the biliary tree:

A. Oral cholecystographic contrast media give good results during acute cholecystitis.
B. Ipodate leaves no radio-opaque residue in the gut.
C. Up to 15 punctures are performed with a fine, flexible needle in percutaneous transhepatic cholangiography (PTC).
D. Erect films are useful in PTC.
E. Contrast containing 350 mg iodine per 100 ml is used at operative cholangiography.

31 In the examination of the biliary tree:

A. It is abnormal for the intramural segment of the bile duct to appear as a gap on T-tube cholangiography.
B. Reflux of contrast along the pancreatic duct during T-tube cholangiography indicates ductal obstruction.
C. 15 ml of contrast should be injected before any films are exposed at operative cholangiography.
D. The upper limit for the diameter of the normal bile duct on radiographs is 14 mm.
E. Stasis of contrast on a post-operative intravenous cholangiogram indicates existing obstruction.

Answers overleaf

30A
FALSE—The gall bladder frequently fails to opacify. This has been shown to be due to the action of bacteria which deconjugate the contrast and permit its reabsorption by the gall bladder itself. Reference *S*, p. 60.

30B
FALSE

30C
FALSE—If the ducts are dilated, then the procedure is best abandoned on failure to enter a bile duct after four needle insertions. Reference *S*, p. 81.

30D
TRUE—They may give the best demonstration of the common bile duct of any films taken. Reference *S*, p. 81.

30E
FALSE—The contrast preferred is one containing 150 mg per 100 ml (e.g. Hypaque 25%). Too high a concentration of iodine will obscure small stones. Reference *S*, p. 76.

31A
FALSE—The intramural segment normally has a narrow lumen or appears as a gap on a T-tube or operative cholangiography. It should not be interpreted as abnormal. Reference *E*, p. 788.

31B
FALSE—This is a common finding in the normal examination. Reference *E*, p. 788.

31C
FALSE—The first film should be taken after the injection of about 3 ml because the terminal portion of the bile duct may otherwise be obscured by contrast in the duodenum. A satisfactory sequence is to take films when 3, 5–8, and 12 ml have been injected. Reference *S*, p. 76.

31D
FALSE—The accepted normal range is 2–10 mm. Reference *E*, p. 787.

31E
TRUE—Distension and over-filling of the hepatic radicles also suggests obstruction. Reference *E*, p. 791.

32 Endoscopic retrograde cholangiopancreatography (ERCP):

A. Is indicated in the investigation of pancreatic pseudocyst.
B. Is contra-indicated in the presence of thoracic aortic aneurysm.
C. Is hazardous in the presence of duodenual diverticula.
D. Requires 8–12 ml to fill the normal pancreatic duct.
E. Has a risk of 1% of causing pancreatitis.

33 In the percutaneous extraction of retained biliary calculi:

A. The optimum time for the procedure is 2 weeks post-operation.
B. The catheter is manipulated to a point distal to a stone in the common bile duct.
C. A Dormia basket is used to capture the stone.
D. If a standard angiographic catheter is used the T-tube is removed prior to insertion of the guide wire.
E. Antibiotic cover is necessary.

Answers overleaf

32A
FALSE—This is a contra-indication to the procedure. If discovered during the procedure, it should not be fully opacified. Antibiotics are given and surgical drainage within 24 hours considered. Reference *S*, p. 87 and p. 92.

32B
TRUE—Reference *S*, p. 87.

32C
FALSE—Although they may make endoscopy difficult.

32D
FALSE—2–5 ml are required. Reference *S*, p. 88.

32E
TRUE—Reference *S*, p. 92.

33A
FALSE—The T-tube is left for 4–6 weeks to allow a good fibrous tract to form before the procedure is attempted. Reference *K*, p. 120.

33B
TRUE—The extraction device can then be advanced to the catheter tip. The catheter is then withdrawn to permit capture of the stone. Reference *K*, p. 121.

33C
TRUE—It should not be advanced beyond the tip of the catheter because of the risk of ductal injury, including perforation. Reference *K*, p. 121.

33D
FALSE—The T-tube is removed after the guide wire is inserted. The catheter is then passed over the guide. Reference *K*, p. 122.

33E
TRUE—A broad-spectrum antibiotic is given for 24 hours before, and for 2–3 days after, the procedure. Reference *K*, p. 121.

34 In arthrography of the knee:

A. The needle should be introduced superior to the patella.
B. The integrity of the cruciates is demonstrated in the AP projection.
C. Ioxoglate is less rapidly absorbed than iothalamate.
D. Adrenaline reduces synovial secretion.
E. 15–20 ml of positive contrast are usually required.

35 In arthrography of the knee:

A. There is no need to aspirate a joint effusion before injection of contrast.
B. Double-contrast is the method of choice for demonstrating cartilage lesions.
C. Double-contrast is the method of choice for evaluating radio-opaque loose bodies.
D. Intra-articular injection of contrast usually causes some pain.
E. Some positive-contrast remains in the normal joint for up to 24 hours.

Answers overleaf

34A
FALSE—The needle is introduced into the patello-femoral joint space, at a point 1 cm posterior to the mid-point of the patella. Either a lateral or medial approach can be used. Reference *S*, p. 307.

34B
FALSE—This may be accomplished in the lateral view with the knee flexed at 60 degrees or more. A film should be taken with the tibia under stress from being drawn anteriorly. Reference *S*, p. 307.

34C
TRUE—Because, being a dimer, ioxoglate has a large molecule and a slower rate of absorption than monomeric compounds such as iothalamate. Ioxoglate is preferred when the procedure is prolonged. Reference *S*, p. 305.

34D
TRUE—0.3 ml of 1 in 1000 adrenaline may be added to the contrast. Reference *S*, p. 305.

34E
FALSE—About 3 ml are injected. Reference *S*, p. 307.

35A
FALSE—It is important that an effusion be aspirated because it will dilute the contrast and also causes bubble formation. Reference *S*, p. 307.

35B
TRUE—Because the method leads to a thin layer of contrast over the cartilage being outlined by air within the joint. Single positive- contrast arthrography is best for determining whether ligaments, tendons or the joint capsule are ruptured. Reference *K*, p. 57.

35C
FALSE—Negative-contrast is best in this situation because contrast will obscure the loose body. Negative-contrast arthrography gives poor film contrast and detail of internal joint structures. Reference *K*, p. 57

35D
FALSE—The injection is painless. If the patient complains of pain, an extra-articular injection should be suspected — in which case, the contrast medium will remain around the needle tip. Reference *K*, p. 61.

35E
FALSE—It is rapidly absorbed. Air, however, remains for 2–3 days The patient should be warned that he will experience some discomfor during this time. Reference *K*, p. 61.

36 In hip arthrography:

A. Sedation or general anaesthesia is required in young children.
B. Fluoroscopy is used to assist needle placement.
C. The anterior (vertical) approach is favoured when there is a hip prosthesis.
D. A small amount of contrast enters the narrow zone of lucency that surrounds the normal prosthesis.
E. Subtraction films should be obtained where there is a prosthesis.

37 In hysterosalpingography:

A. Pethidine is suitable for premedication.
B. Urografin 370 is a suitable contrast.
C. The procedure is abandoned if venous intravasation occurs.
D. The scar of previous caesarian section is demonstrated on frontal films.
E. Uterine malignancy is a contra-indication to the procedure.

Answers overleaf

36A
TRUE—Reference *S*, p. 308.

36B
TRUE—Reference *K*, p. 78.

36C
FALSE—An anterolateral approach is preferred because the prosthesis obscures the metallic needle. Reference *K*, p. 79.

36D
FALSE—This suggests that loosening of the prosthesis has occurred. Reference *K*, p. 78.

36E
TRUE—Because of the difficulty in distinguishing contrast from the radio-opaque cement. Reference *K*, p. 79.

37A
FALSE—It stimulates smooth muscle. This may result in difficulty in filling the tubes. Reference *S*, p. 245.

37B
TRUE—Because of its high viscosity at room temperature. Reference *S*, p. 248.

37C
FALSE—The incidence of intravasation is 0.6–3.7%. It is of no significance. The cannula is repositioned and a successful examination usually obtained. Reference *S*, p. 249.

37D
FALSE—A lateral view is required. The uterus is carrot shaped in this projection. Reference *S*, p. 248.

37E
FALSE—It may be used to evaluate the extent of endometrial carcinoma. Dissemination of tumour cells by the technique is not known to occur. Reference *S*, p. 244.

38 In lymphography:

A. The thoracic duct cannot normally be demonstrated.
B. The injection is made at a rate of about 15 ml per hour.
C. The injection is stopped if there is marked obstruction.
D. A 24 gauge needle is used to cannulate the lymphatics.
E. Follow-up films add no diagnostic information in patients with malignant disease.

39 In lymphography:

A. Small veins may be mistaken for a lymphatic.
B. The contrast medium should be seen as globules on a radiograph of the calf.
C. Blood staining of the sputum in the week after injection usually indicates that a pulmonary oil embolus has occurred.
D. Cerebral oil embolus is a rare but usually fatal complication.
E. 24-hour films are taken to demonstrate the lymphatic vessels.

Answers overleaf

38A

FALSE—It will be opacified on films of the chest taken at the end of the procedure. Reference *J*, p. 286.

38B

FALSE—The maximum desirable rate is 10 ml per hour. Faster injection rates than this will cause extravasation. Reference *J*, p. 285.

38C

TRUE—The injection should also be stopped on identifying a lymphatico-venous connection. Reference *S*, p. 187.

38D

FALSE—27–30 gauge needles are used. Reference *J*, p. 280.

38E

FALSE—They are of great importance. The contrast remains in the nodes for up to a year or more in diagnostic amounts. This permits assessment of the effect of treatment and may give added information over the immediate and 24-hour films. Reference *S*, p. 189.

39A

TRUE—Because of this, it is advisable to take a radiograph of the calf at an early stage of the injection. Reference *S*, p. 186.

39B

FALSE—Globulation occurs when Lipiodol is injected intravenously. It has been described as the 'caviare sign'. Reference *S*, p. 186.

39C

FALSE—Slight blood staining of the sputum occurs in about one-fifth of patients between 3 and 10 days after injection. It is thought to result from the breakdown of the oily contrast into fatty acids in the lungs. Reference *S*, p. 190.

39D

FALSE—In a series of 10 000, two cases of cerebral oil emboli were recorded. Both patients recovered completely. Reference *S*, p. 190.

39E

FALSE—The lymphatic vessels are devoid of contrast at 24 hours. The films at this time show the nodes. Reference *S*, p. 188.

40 In lymphography:

A. The procedure may be performed if the patient is receiving a course of radiotherapy to the chest.
B. Severe emphysema is a contra-indication to the procedure.
C. The injection is stopped when the cisterna chyli is seen.
D. Ideally, 20 ml Lipiodol is used in each leg.
E. The internal iliac nodes are usually demonstrated.

41 In the normal pedal lymphangiogram:

A. The cisterna chyli is usually demonstrated as a distinct sac at the level of L2.
B. The left chain of lumbar lymph nodes usually extends higher than the right.
C. Lymphatics do not cross between the lumbar trunks.
D. A gap in the lumbar lymph trunk on the right is abnormal
E. The lumbar nodes may normally extend laterally beyond the tips of the transverse processes.

Answers overleaf

40A

FALSE—It is unsafe in this situation because of the risk of cerebral oil embolus. Reference *J*, p. 279.

40B

TRUE—Because there is depression of lung function after the injection of contrast as the oil is filtered by the pulmonary capillaries. Reference *S*, p. 183.

40C

FALSE—The injection is stopped when the contrast medium has reached the level of L4. Reference *S*, p. 188.

40D

FALSE—A maximum of 8 ml is used per side. Reference *S*, p. 188.

40E

FALSE—These nodes receive lymph from pelvic structures, but not the lower limbs.

41A

FALSE—It is intermittently demonstrated and then is usually seen as a plexus of vessels. Reference: Jackson, B. T. and Kinmonth, J. B. The normal lymphographic appearances of the lumbar lymphatics. *Clinical Radiology*; **25**:175–86 (1974).

41B

TRUE—In 51% of cases it extends to a higher vertebral level than the right or the mid chain. The right reaches a higher level in 17% of cases. Reference: *Clinical Radiology*; **25**:175–86 (1974).

41C

FALSE—Cross-over occurs in 45% of lymphangiograms. Cross-over from right to left occurs twice as commonly as in the reverse direction, which presumably accounts for the finding of metastases from right gonadal tumours in the left lumbar nodes in a significant number of patients. Reference: Jackson, B. T. and Kinmonth, J. B. Lumbar lymphatic crossover. *Clinical Radiology*; **25**:187–93 (1974).

41D

FALSE—It is associated with a right lower lumbar bypass vessel, usually at the L3/4 level. In contrast, the left lumbar chain is always continuous. Reference: *Clinical Radiology*; **25**:187–93 (1974).

41E

FALSE—If they do, then they are displaced. Reference: *Clinical Radiology*; **25**:187–93 (1974).

42 Hepatic oil embolism following lymphography:

A. Occurs as a result of lymphaticoportal anastomoses.
B. May occur when the nodes are normal.
C. May appear as irregular streaks of increased attenuation on CT.
D. Causes a permanent change in the radiological appearance of the liver parenchyma.
E. Tends to occur in the left lobe with sparing of the right lobe.

43 In sialography:

A. The parotid duct opens opposite the upper canine.
B. The duct of the parotid gland is approximately 6 cm in length.
C. The injection may be made via gravity and a reservoir of contrast some 70 cm above the patient's head.
D. The success of the procedure in examining the parotid depends on the rapid injection of 2–3 ml of contrast.
E. The sublingual ducts may open into the submaxillary duct.

Answers overleaf

42A

TRUE—Reference: Silverstone, E. J., *et al*. The CT appearances of hepatic oil embolism following lymphography. *British Journal of Radiology*; **57**:779–83 (1984).

42B

FALSE—The nodes must be diseased, because the lymphatico-venous connections do not open up unless there is obstruction to the lymphatics. Reference: *British Journal of Radiology*; **57**:779–83 (1984).

42C

TRUE—This should not be confused with metastatic disease. The presence of lymphatic opacification or, rarely, free intraperitoneal contrast will suggest the correct diagnosis. Reference: *British Journal of Radiology*; **57**:779–83 (1984).

42D

FALSE—The oil disperses. Reference: *British Journal of Radiology*; **57**:779–83 (1984).

42E

FALSE—The left lobe is spared. This may be due to the heavy oil gravitating to the more inferiorly placed right portal vein. Reference: *British Journal of Radiology*; **57**:779–83 (1984).

43A

FALSE—It opens opposite the second upper molar. Reference *S*, p. 5.

43B

TRUE—Reference *H*, p. 766.

43C

TRUE—The secreting pressure of the gland lies between 54 and 76 cm of water; hence, the reservoir has to be elevated to a height of about 70 cm in order to exceed this. Reference *S*, p. 8.

43D

FALSE—The injection should be made very slowly. In the healthy gland, 0.5–0.75 ml of contrast is often adequate. Too fast an injection causes pain. The maximum amount that should be injected is 2 ml at one time. Reference *S*, p. 6.

43E

TRUE—So that they may be injected in error. Reference *H*, p. 766.

44 In the investigation of facial structures:

A. The inferior canaliculus of the lacrimal system has a vertical and a horizontal component.
B. Ioxaglate is preferred for dacrocystography.
C. ^{99m}Tc-labelled DTPA is used for the technique of lacrimal scintillography.
D. Delayed films are obtained in sialography.
E. The cannula may be removed from the parotid duct before exposing films when using water-soluble contrast.

45 In bronchography:

A. Propyliodone is the contrast of choice.
B. 1 ml of contrast per year of age per side is required in children of normal size.
C. Premedication is unnecessary.
D. The use of lignocaine is hazardous only when it is given in doses of 800 mg or more.
E. Some contrast may be detected in the bronchi for up to 3 weeks.

Answers overleaf

44A
TRUE—The vertical component is about 2 mm long, whilst the horizontal part is 7 mm or so in length. Reference *J*, p. 120.

44B
FALSE—Lipiodol is the contrast of choice. About 2 ml is injected. Reference *S*, p. 301.

44C
FALSE—Tc-labelled sulphur colloid is used. Reference *Z2*, p. 115.

44D
TRUE—To assess the clearing of contrast from the gland, films are exposed after a sialogue (e.g. a slice of lemon) has been sucked by the patient. Reference *S*, p. 8.

44E
FALSE—Water-soluble contrast is used by some radiologists. It must have a high iodine concentration. Because of its relatively low viscosity, the cannula must be left in the duct when taking films, or significant leaking of contrast out of the duct will occur. Reference *S*, p. 6.

45A
TRUE—Propyliodone (Dionosil) is available either as a suspension in arachis oil or as an aqueous suspension. The latter gives better coating of the bronchial mucosa and may also be diluted. Reference *S*, p. 202.

45B
TRUE—With an additional 1–3 ml if there is plain film evidence of bronchiectasis. Reference *J*, p. 147.

45C
FALSE—It is an unpleasant procedure which requires both a sedative and an agent for reducing bronchial secretions. Reference *S*, p. 202.

45D
FALSE—Convulsions and cardiorespiratory problems occur when 200 mg or more is given. Reference *S*, p. 202.

45E
FALSE—It is usually entirely expectorated within 2 days. Reference *S*, p. 203.

46 In bronchography:

A. Oily contrast is less irritant than aqueous contrast.
B. Aqueous contrast gives better filling of small bronchi than oily contrast.
C. Asthma is a contra-indication to the procedure.
D. The catheter is placed in the right main bronchus for examination of the right lung.
E. Oily contrast is not used with a fibre-optic bronchoscope.

47 In fluoroscopy of the chest:

A. The left leaf of the diaphragm usually moves more than the right.
B. Sniffing causes upward movement of the diaphragm.
C. The dependent leaf of the diaphragm has less mobility in the decubitus patient.
D. Vascular structures diminish in size during the Valsalva manoeuvre.
E. Areas of calcification within the heart can be demonstrated.

Answers overleaf

46A
TRUE—Reference *J*, p. 134.

46B
FALSE—Oily contrast gives better peripheral filling. Reference *S*, p. 202.

46C
TRUE—Because the procedure may provoke an attack. Reference *S*, p. 202.

46D
FALSE—It is placed in the intermediate bronchus. Reference *S*, p. 204.

46E
TRUE—Because it cannot be removed from the bronchoscope.

47A
TRUE—Reference *W*, p. 435.

47B
FALSE—The diaphragm normally moves downwards. An upward movement is paradoxical and may be seen in paralysis. Reference *W*, p. 435.

47C
FALSE—It has greater mobility and usually lies high in the chest. Reference *W*, p. 435.

47D
TRUE—This may help to distinguish them from non-vascular structures such as enlarged nodes. Reference *W*, p. 7.

47E
TRUE—And their exact site determined. Reference *H*, p. 720.

48 In tomography of the paranasal sinuses and orbits, the radiation dose to the eyes is reduced by:

A. Using rare-earth screens rather than calcium tungstate screens.
B. Use of the AP position.
C. Correct selection of plane of tomographic cut.
D. The use, in practice, of eye shields.
E. Hypocycloidal rather than linear movement.

Answers overleaf

48A

TRUE—Reference: Eddlestone, B., *et al.* Eye dose measurements using conventional and rare earth screens during tomography of the paranasal sinuses. *British Journal of Radiology*; **50**:266–70 (1977).

48B

FALSE—A 98% reduction in dose to the eyes can be obtained by use of the PA position: e.g. for Agfa Gevaert MR 400 (blue-emitting rare earth) screens and Kodak RP 56 film, the dose measured was 400 and 8 mrad in the AP and PA positions, respectively. Reference: *British Journal of Radiology*; **50**:266–70 (1977).

48C

TRUE—By keeping the number of exposures to a minimum.

48D

FALSE—Eye shields, although they halve the dose to the eyes in tomography of the middle ear, cause blurring of the image in the orbito-ethmoidal region. They are not, therefore, practicable. Reference: *British Journal of Radiology*; **50**:266–70 (1977).

48E

FALSE—In Eddlestone's study, the average dose for linear tomography was 26.4 mrad per cut, and for hypocycloidal, 33.5 mrad per cut. Reference: *British Journal of Radiology*; **50**:266–70 (1977).

49 Concerning the hips and pelvis:

A. The AP view of the hip is centred 2 cm below the midpoint of the inguinal ligament.
B. The angle of anteversion of the femoral neck on the femoral shaft is 15–20 degrees in adults.
C. In the 'von Rosen' position the legs are abducted 25 degrees from the midline.
D. In the 'von Rosen' position the legs are internally rotated.
E. The acetabular angle (the slope of the acetabulum to the horizontal) is normally about 40 degrees in a child of 6 months.

Answers overleaf

49A

TRUE—Reference *R*, p. 133 Figs 497–8. The inguinal ligament extends from the anterior superior iliac spine to the pubic tubercle.

49B

FALSE—It is normally about 8 degrees. Reference *H*, p. 134 (Table 5-1).

49C

FALSE—This view is used for demonstrating congenital dislocation of the hip. In the normal pelvis, a line drawn through the femoral shaft will be directed to the upper edge of the bony acetabular wall. In congenital dislocation, the line of the femoral shaft will point to the anterior superior iliac spine. At least 45 degrees of abduction is essential if the view is not to give misleading results. Reference *H*, p. 145.

49D

TRUE—Reference *H*, p. 145.

49E

FALSE—The angle is normally no more than 34 degrees in a child aged between 3 and 12 months. Before this age, the normal range is very wide. The angle is of use in assessing congenital dislocation of the hip. Reference *H*, p. 144.

50 In plain abdominal radiography:

A. A short exposure time is unnecessary.
B. The lower border of the cassette should be positioned at the level of the symphysis pubis.
C. The erect abdominal film is more likely to show free subdiaphragmatic air than an erect chest film.
D. As little as 1 ml of free intraperitoneal air may be demonstrated.
E. The injection of 50 ml of air via a nasogastric tube may assist in the diagnosis of a perforation.

51 The following projections are appropriate:

A. A right posterior oblique 15–25 degrees for the demonstration of the left sacroiliac joint.
B. The AP oblique projection of the wrist for optimal demonstration of the pisiform.
C. The left posterior oblique 25 degrees to demonstrate the right glenohumeral joint.
D. The AP knee for optimal frontal demonstration of the patella.
E. A left posterior oblique 45 degrees for visualization of the left pars interarticularis.

Answers overleaf

50A
FALSE—A short exposure time is used so that movement blur does not affect the image. Ideally, it should not exceed 0.08 seconds. Reference *S*, p. 376.

50B
FALSE—The cassette should be placed below the symphysis pubis, because otherwise the obliquity of the rays will project the pubis off the film. Reference *S*, p. 376.

50C
FALSE—Because of the lower exposure used, and because the centring point is more favourable, the chest radiograph is superior to the erect film of the abdomen in detecting free subdiaphragmatic air. Reference: Miller, R. E. and Nelson, S. W. The roentgenologic demonstration of tiny amounts of free intraperitoneal gas: experimental and clinical studies. *Am. J. Roent*; **112**:574–85 (1971).

50D
TRUE—Miller and Nelson showed that this was possible. The best method for showing free gas is to lie the patient in the left lateral decubitus position for at least 10 minutes prior to performing an erect film of the chest. Reference: *Am. J. Roent*; **112**:574–85 (1971).

50E
TRUE—Reference *S*, p. 11.

51A
TRUE—Reference *R*, p. 166.

51B
TRUE—The best view of the pisiform is obtained by this projection. Reference *R*, p. 15 (Fig. 50).

51C
FALSE—This position would be suitable for showing the left glenohumeral joint. Reference *R*, p. 63.

51D
FALSE—It is best done PA so as to bring the patella close to the film and thereby to reduce magnification and geometric unsharpness (Reference *H*, p. 164). A short focus-to-film distance may be used to blur the femoral condyles. It is important to support the patient's thigh and ankle for comfort.

51E
TRUE—The opposite side to the sacroiliac joint demonstrated. Reference *H*, p. 130.

52 In the radiography of the cervical spine:

A. No tube angulation is required in the AP view provided that the canthomeatal line (CML) is at 90 degrees to the film.
B. The intervertebral foramina nearer the film are seen in the AP oblique projection.
C. Tomography is often essential when there is an injury to the axis.
D. The AP view is done first in the injured, stretchered patient.
E. A long focus-to-film distance is required for the lateral projection.

Answers overleaf

52A

FALSE—The CML is elevated above the horizontal so as to superimpose mandible and occiput and display as much of the cervical vertebrae as possible. The tube is angled 5–10 degrees cephalad. Reference *R*, p. 182.

52B

FALSE—The foramina nearer the tube are seen (Reference *R*, p. 188). Whether performed AP or PA, the foramina demonstrated are those away from the side to which the patient is looking.

52C

TRUE—When there is a fracture of the dens and there is difficulty in positioning the head so that there is no superimposition of other structures, tomography will usually provide a clear view of the area. Reference *R*, p. 181.

52D

FALSE—The lateral projection is performed first using a horizontal beam. It is viewed before going onto the AP projection. Reference *R*, p. 186.

52E

TRUE—The long object-to-film distance tends to cause a loss of definition, especially if a broad focus is used. A long focus-to-film distance is employed to reduce magnification and loss of definition. Reference *R*, p. 184.

53 Patient movement during an exposure may be usefully employed in:

A. The AP view of the lumbar spine.
B. The PA view of the scapula.
C. The lateral oblique view of the temporomandibular joints.
D. The AP view of the cervical spine.
E. The prone oblique view of the sternum.

54 The lordotic AP projection of the chest is useful in evaluating:

A. An apical lesion.
B. The middle lobe.
C. Pleural effusions.
D. Fluid in the oblique fissure.
E. The carina.

Answers overleaf

53A
TRUE—A long exposure in this situation may help to blur out the unwanted image of bowel gas. Reference *R*, p. 204.

53B
TRUE—The shadows of the ribs are blurred when the patient breathes gently and smoothly during a long exposure of about 5 seconds. Reference *R*, p. 64.

53C
FALSE—Views are taken with the mouth open and closed. Reference *R*, p. 322.

53D
TRUE—The mandible may be blurred out usefully by the patient opening and closing his mouth during a prolonged exposure. All the cervical vertebrae can then be seen on a single exposure. Reference *R*, p. 184.

53E
TRUE—The rib shadows are blurred out (Reference *R*, p. 237). The lateral view of the dorsal spine also makes use of patient movement during an exposure.

54A
TRUE—The projection may help when the apices of the lung are obscured on the standard PA film by ribs or clavicle. Reference *E*, p. 235.

54B
TRUE—This is because the longest axis of the lobe takes up a position that is more in line with the X-ray. Reference *E*, p. 235.

54C
FALSE—A lateral decubitus film is useful for demonstrating effusions. Reference *E*, p. 236.

54D
TRUE—The fissure is at less of an oblique angle to the X-ray in this projection. Reference *E*, p. 235.

54E
FALSE—An over-penetrated film or tomography are useful. Reference *E*, p. 236 and 238.

55 The following are features of the air-gap technique for radiography of the chest:

A. The dose of radiation to the skin is higher than with conventional radiography.
B. Good definition of mediastinal structures.
C. Good definition of soft pulmonary shadows.
D. Wide exposure latitude.
E. The use of selective filters.

56 In radiography of the chest:

A. A pleural effusion consisting of 5–10 ml of fluid can be seen in a lateral decubitus position.
B. Lower lobe disease is best seen in the lordotic projection.
C. Only the posterior portion of the left hemidiaphragm is seen on the lateral projection.
D. The posterior wall of the bronchus intermedius can usually be seen on a lateral film.
E. Heart size does not usually increase by more than 1.5 cm in consecutive films.

Answers overleaf

55A
FALSE—It is lower because the X-ray beam used has a higher peak energy (120 kVp or more). Reference *H*, p. 650.

55B
TRUE—Reference *H*, p. 650.

55C
FALSE—Reference *H*, p. 650.

55D
TRUE

55E
TRUE—These are necessary because of the wide range of density between mediastinum and lung. Reference *Z*3, p. 747.

56A
TRUE—This was shown by Moskowitz *et al.* when they took films of a corpse in the lateral decubitus position after they had injected the pleural cavity with small amounts of fluid. Reference: Moskowitz, H., *et al.* Roentgen visualization of minute pleural effusion: an experimental study to determine the minimum amount of pleural fluid visible on a radiograph. *Radiology*; **109**:33–5 (1973).

56B
FALSE

56C
TRUE—This is one of the signs used to differentiate the leaves of the diaphragm on the lateral film. Reference *N*, 22.3 p. 617.

56D
TRUE—It forms a radiodense strip 0.5–3.0 mm wide between the air in the bronchus and the lung in the azygo-oesophageal recess. It can be seen in most lateral films, and well in about 55%. It is always well demonstrated by CT. A varied number of pathological conditions can cause the strip to be thickened. Reference: Webb, W. R., *et al.* Posterior wall of the bronchus intermedius: radiographic-CT correlation. *Am. J. Roent*; **142**:907–11 (1984).

56E
TRUE—Although in two 'normal' patients in a series of 100, the heart was 2 and 3 cm larger. Reference *Z*4.

57 In pelvimetry:

A. A kVp of 60–70 should be used.
B. The sagittal (AP) diameter of the inlet normally measures 10–10.5 cm.
C. The central beam is directed at the symphysis pubis in the AP view.
D. The outlet diameter increases during late pregnancy.
E. The bispinous diameter is normally greater than 10 cm.

Answers overleaf

57A

FALSE—A high kVp of 100–120 is used to limit the radiation dose. Reference *Z*5.

57B

FALSE—The mean value is 11.6 cm. Contraction exists when the diameter is less than 10.5 cm. Reference *Z*5.

57C

FALSE—The centring point is 2 cm above the symphysis pubis. Reference *Z*5.

57D

TRUE—Because of relaxation of the symphysis pubis and rotation of the sacroiliac joints. The measurement may increase by 1–1.75 cm. It is argued that pelvimetry should be performed at the onset of labour to take this into account. Reference *Z*5.

57E

TRUE—If it is less than 10 cm it indicates contraction. Reference *Z*5.

58 The following are absolutely or relatively contra-indicated:

A. Barium follow-through in suspected small-bowel obstruction.
B. Intravenous cholangiography when oral cholecystography has failed 24 hours previously.
C. Hysterosalpingography performed in the mid-part of the menstrual cycle.
D. Percutaneous transhepatic cholangiography in a patient with cholestatic jaundice.
E. Pulmonary angiography when the end-diastolic pulmonary pressures are greater than 20 mm Hg.

59 In abdominal ultrasound:

A. The intrahepatic branches of the hepatic artery are not generally seen.
B. Portal veins are identified by the high-intensity echoes around them.
C. The normal pancreatic duct cannot be seen.
D. Free blood can be distinguished from ascites.
E. The AP diameter of the normal pancreas is 1–3 cm.

Answers overleaf

58A
FALSE—The small intestine secretes fluid which dilutes the barium so that there is no realistic danger of impaction. Barium is advantageous to conventional water-soluble contrast because of its greater density and because it has fewer side effects. Reference *S*, p. 22.

58B
TRUE—In this situation, there is a greater incidence of both major and minor reactions, and poor visualization of the ducts is more likely. Reference: Finby, N. and Blasberg, G. A note on the blocking of hepatic excretion during cholangiographic study. *Gastroenterology*; **46**:276–7 (1964).

58C
FALSE—This is a good time to perform the examination because there is less likelihood of cornual spasm or intravasation of contrast. Reference *S*, p. 245.

58D
FALSE—This procedure is used to make the distinction between a cholestatic jaundice and an extrahepatic obstruction. Reference *S*, p. 80.

58E
TRUE—There were three deaths in a series of 1350 pulmonary angiograms. These patients all had raised end-diastolic pulmonary pressures (over 20 mm Hg). The deaths occurred 1–2 hours after the injection of contrast. Although catheterization had been uneventful, the injection of contrast had resulted in a drop in the systemic arterial pressure and eventually death in all three patients. Reference: Mills, S. R., *et al*. The incidence, etiologies and avoidance of complications of pulmonary angiography in a large series. *Radiology*; **136**:295–9 (1980).

59A
TRUE—Reference *E*, p. 1350.

59B
TRUE—Reference *T*, p. 81.

59C
FALSE—Segments of it may be seen and normally measure no more than 3 mm in diameter. Reference *T*, p. 88.

59D
FALSE—Reference *E*, p. 1357.

59E
TRUE—The pancreas has a crescenteric shape on transverse section. Reference *E*, p. 1352.

60 In the technique of ultrasound:

A. Subcutaneous fat may produce reverberation echoes.
B. Careful selection of the depth of a water bath is unnecessary.
C. Areas of low attenuation give rise to an artefactual accentuation of echoes from deeper structures.
D. Water baths are not indicated in scanning neonates.
E. Olive oil cannot be used as the coupling fluid.

61 At ultrasound examination of the abdomen:

A. The hepatic artery is seen.
B. The spleen is usually well seen on a scan made through the anterior abdominal wall.
C. The spiral valve of the gall bladder causes a distal acoustic shadow.
D. The renal pyramids may be seen as separate structures.
E. The adrenal glands are more reliably imaged than with CT.

Answers overleaf

60A
TRUE—And this may obscure anterior structures such as the anterior bladder wall. Reference *T*, p. 52.

60B
FALSE—The depth must be greater than that of the structure being examined. If it is less than this, any reverberations between the transducer and the bath bottom will be displayed over the area of interest. Reference *T*, p. 52.

60C
TRUE—The echoes received from liver beyond a cyst or the gall bladder may be enhanced in this way. The artefact results from time gain compensation. Reference *T*, p. 52.

60D
FALSE—They may be helpful because their warmth may serve to comfort the child and because they insulate the child from the movements of the transducer. Reference *T*, p. 50.

60E
FALSE—It is perfectly adequate. Paraffin oil, which is also suitable, is advocated by some and has the advantage of low cost. Oils are sticky so that patient preference is for the more easily removed hypoallergenic gels. Reference *T*, p. 54.

61A
TRUE—With the splenic artery, it is seen on a transverse section branching from the coeliac axis in a 'seagull' pattern. Reference *F*, p. 79.

61B
FALSE—Visualization of the spleen frequently requires scanning in the lower intercostal spaces (e.g. the tenth). It may help to lie the patient on his right side. By this means, a scan along the length of the spleen is obtained. This is normally not greater than 12 cm. Reference *T*, p. 130.

61C
TRUE—Which should not be confused with a calculus. Reference *T*, p. 90.

61D
TRUE—Reference *T*, p. 101.

61E
FALSE

62 In the use of ultrasound:

A. The hepatic veins have poorly echogenic walls.
B. The renal parenchyma appears as dense as that of liver.
C. The renal hilum is echo free.
D. The bile duct normally measures 6–9 mm in diameter.
E. The gall bladder is best examined after the patient has had a fatty meal.

63 In fetal ultrasound:

A. Pulsations of the heart are first seen at 7 weeks with a real-time scanner.
B. The four-chamber view of the heart is obtained with a scan at 60 degrees to the long axis of the fetus.
C. The gestation sac is first detected at about 6 weeks after the last menstrual period (LMP).
D. The umbilical vein can be usually demonstrated.
E. Dense echoes are obtained from the mid-line of the fetal skull when intrauterine death has occurred.

Answers overleaf

62A
TRUE—A feature that helps to identify them. Reference *T*, p. 81.

62B
FALSE—It appears less dense than liver. Reference *T*, p. 98 (Fig. 9.1).

62C
FALSE—It is echo dense. The echoes probably emanate from renal vessels. Reference *T*, p. 101.

62D
FALSE—It should not normally measure more than 5 mm in diameter. Reference *T*, p. 101.

62E
FALSE—It is essential that the patient is adequately fasted so as to distend the gall bladder as much as possible. The contractility of the organ can be subsequently assessed by giving the patient a fatty meal. Reference *T*, p. 89.

63A
TRUE—Reference *M*, p. 410.

63B
FALSE—It is achieved with a transverse scan of the thorax. Reference *M*, p. 508.

63C
TRUE—Reference *T*, p. 58.

63D
TRUE—Measurements of fetal abdominal circumference made at this level can be extrapolated to give an estimate of fetal weight. Reference: Campbell, S. and Wilkin, D. Ultrasonic measurement of fetal abdomen circumference in the estimation of fetal weight. *British Journal of Obstetrics and Gynaecology*; **82**:689–97 (1975).

63E
FALSE—The mid-line echoes disappear in fetal death. Other signs of intrauterine death include the loss of fetal heart motion, oedema of the skin (giving a double outline to the head and a halo of echoes around the body), and bizarre shape of the head. Reference *F*, p. 29.

64 The biparietal diameter (BPD) of the fetal skull:

A. Is measured from the 7th week after the LMP.
B. Is measured at the level of the cavum of the septum pellucidum.
C. Is normally greater than 70 mm at 20 weeks.
D. Is normally 90 mm at term.
E. Gives a less accurate estimate of fetal maturity in the third trimester than earlier in pregnancy.

65 In the obstetric patient;

A. The fetus is identified radiographically at about 10 weeks after the LMP.
B. The dilatation of the calices seen at intravenous urography during pregnancy usually resolves at about 4 weeks post partum.
C. The crown–rump length is accurate in assessing fetal age up to the 20th week of pregnancy.
D. The crown–lump length at 10 weeks is 33 mm.
E. A crown–rump length of 27 mm is compatible with a menstrual age of 8 weeks.

Answers overleaf

64A
FALSE—The fetal head is measurable from about the 12th week of pregnancy. Reference *T*, p. 64.

64B
TRUE—Which is also the level of the thalamus and third ventricle. Reference *M*, p. 427.

64C
FALSE—The mean BPD at this time is 50.2 mm. Mean measurements of 70 mm or more are obtained in normal pregnancies after 26 weeks. Reference: Campbell, S. and Newman, G. B. Growth of the fetal biparietal diameter during normal pregnancy. *Journal of Obstetrics and Gynaecology of the British Commonwealth*; **78**:513–9 (1971).

64D
FALSE—The mean BPD at term is 98.1 mm. Reference: *Journal of Obstetrics and Gynaecology of the British Commonwealth*; **78**:513–9 (1971).

64E
TRUE—Because the rate of growth is slower and because of moulding of the fetal head late in pregnancy. Reference *M*, p. 427.

65A
FALSE—It usually becomes visible at 16 weeks. Reference *E*, p. 919.

65B
FALSE—It resolves at about 10–12 weeks. Reference *E*, p. 919.

65C
FALSE—It becomes inaccurate after 12 weeks because of flexion of the fetal spine. Reference *M*, p. 423.

65D
TRUE—Reference: Robinson, H. P. and Fleming, J. E. E. A critical evaluation of sonar 'crown–rump length' measurements. *British Journal of Obstetrics and Gynaecology*; **82**:702–10 (1975).

65E
FALSE—It is consistent with a pregnancy of 9 weeks and 3 days. At 8 weeks, the mean ($\pm$SD) crown–rump length is 17 $\pm$ 4.9 mm. Reference: *British Journal of Obstetrics and Gynaecology*; **82**:702–10 (1975).

66 In pelvic and fetal ultrasound:

A. Correctly sited intra-uterine contraceptive devices are seen.
B. A 'cavitary echo' is seen in the midline of the non-pregnant uterus.
C. Femur length is not a reliable indicator of fetal age.
D. The chorionic plate is not normally visible.
E. The diagnosis of placenta praevia is made in the second trimester.

67 In ultrasonic scanning of ovarian follicles:

A. The right ovary is more commonly undetectable than the left.
B. Follicle size prior to ovulation is normally 22–28 mm.
C. The cumulus oophorous is detectable within the developing follicle.
D. Internal echoes within a full-size follicle indicates that ovulation has failed.
E. The endometrium appears as a ring shadow after ovulation.

Answers overleaf

66A
TRUE—The use of ultrasound is a cost-effective and safe way of checking on their correct placement. Reference *T*, p. 56.

66B
TRUE—It is an echo produced by the contact of the endometrial surfaces. Reference *T*, p. 56.

66C
FALSE—It is at least as reliable as measurement of the BPD. Reference *M*, p. 428.

66D
FALSE—It may be seen as an echogenic line. Reference *T*, p. 67.

66E
FALSE—It should not be diagnosed until at least 32 weeks because the lower uterine segment is not fully developed before this. Commonly, a placenta that extends to the cervical os is seen to migrate out of the lower uterine segment in the third trimester. Reference *T*, p. 68.

67A
FALSE—The left is not seen more often. This is because it is easily covered by the sigmoid colon. Reference *M*, p. 604.

67B
FALSE—The follicle has a diameter of 18–24 mm at the time of ovulation with a mean of 20.2 mm. Reference *M*, p. 607.

67C
TRUE—It is a sign of impending ovulation. Reference *M*, p. 610.

67D
FALSE—It is one of the signs that ovulation has occurred. Reference *M*, p. 611.

67E
TRUE—Reference *M*, p. 614.

68 In water-soluble contrast myelography via a lumbar puncture:

A. The L1/2 interspace is usually used.
B. An extra-arachnoid injection is more likely to occur if the puncture is performed with the patient erect.
C. Iohexol causes a significant change in electroencephalogram (EEG) activity in 50% of patients.
D. The neck is flexed to prevent dispersal of contrast when examining the cervical region.
E. The incidence of side-effects is not reduced by 24 hours bed rest following the procedure.

69 In cerebral angiography:

A. Only the anterior wall of the common carotid artery is punctured in the direct technique of carotid angiography.
B. 6 ml iopamidol 300 at 4 ml s^{-1} is suitable for vertebral angiography.
C. Direct vertebral puncture is best performed with a short bevel needle.
D. Direct puncture of the vertebral artery is performed with the patient's head extended and the carotid artery displaced laterally.
E. Cortical blindness is a complication of carotid angiography.

Answers overleaf

68A
FALSE—The L3/4 interspace is chosen. Reference *S*, p. 266.

68B
FALSE—This is more likely to occur in a decubitus position. This is because the lumbar arachnoid sac is distended in the erect position which makes the successful puncture easier to achieve. Reference *S*, p. 266.

68C
FALSE—No significant change is seen in EEG activity in patients undergoing iohexol myelography. Reference: Kendall, B. and Stevens, J. Cervical myelography with iohexol. *British Journal of Radiology*; **57**:785–7 (1984).

68D
FALSE—Extension of the neck is of prime importance if dispersal of the bolus of contrast is to be avoided. This is because the cervical lordosis acts to pool the contrast. Reference *S*, p. 273.

68E
TRUE—Reference: MacPherson, P. and Teasdale, E. Radiculography with non-ionic contrast medium: routine bedrest is unnecessary. *Clincial Radiology*; **35**:287–8 (1984).

69A
FALSE—The artery is transfixed by puncture of its anterior and posterior walls. The needle is then withdrawn into the lumen. Reference *S*, p. 286.

69B
TRUE—Reference *S*, p. 108.

69C
FALSE—A needle with a blocked tip and side hole is preferred because of the small lumen of the vertebral arteries. Reference *S*, p. 288.

69D
TRUE—The artery is punctured in the mid-cervical region as it passes between the transverse foramina. Reference *S*, p. 288.

69E
FALSE—It complicates vertebral angiography, is usually transient, and is thought to be a toxic effect. Reference *S*, p. 290.

70 The window level of a CT scan:

A. Refers to the range of attenuation values on the grey scale.
B. Should be at, or near to, the attenuation value of the tissue being displayed.
C. Should be 100 for scans of the mediastinum.
D. Should be at the end of the negative scale for images of the lung fields.
E. Has no effect on the measured size of a lesion.

71 In the use of contrast in CT:

A. Bowel need not be opacified when scanning the pancreas.
B. Barium is contra-indicated.
C. An infusion of intravenous contrast is required for maximal enhancement of vascular structures.
D. Oral doses given at two separate times are needed to opacify the gut on abdominal scans.
E. The cephalic vein is preferred for the rapid injection of a bolus of contrast in the arm.

Answers overleaf

70A
FALSE—The range of values is the window width. The midpoint on the grey scale is the window level. Reference *Q*, p. 13.

70B
TRUE—Reference *Q*, p. 13.

70C
FALSE—It should be at zero. Reference *Q*, p. 14.

70D
TRUE—Reference *Q*, p. 15.

70E
FALSE—It has some effect because of partial volume averaging. This is minimized by setting the window level halfway between the lesion density and the density of the background. Reference *Q*, p. 15.

71A
FALSE—Bowel opacification is essential. Bowel that has not been opacified frequently simulates a mass. Reference *Q*, p. 16.

71B
FALSE—Low-density barium (1.5% weight by volume) is available for CT scanning and is probably the contrast of choice in the alimentary tract. Reference *Q*, p. 16.

71C
FALSE—A bolus is needed to give maximal vascular enhancement. Reference *Q*, p. 17.

71D
TRUE—Contrast given 1 hour before will opacify the more distal bowel whereas the proximal bowel will be well opacified by contrast given 15 minutes before scanning. Reference *Q*, p. 17.

71E
FALSE—The median cubital or basilic vein is chosen because of the more direct route to the superior vena cava and because it is not obstructed by the over-the-head position adopted by the arm during a scan. Reference *Q*, p. 18.

72 In a CT scan of the brain using a CT number scale of 2000:

A. White matter has a higher CT number than grey matter.
B. Clotted blood has a density of 50–80 units.
C. Scans are generally made parallel to the canthomeatal line.
D. The skin dose to the patient is about 5 rad for a completed scan.
E. Intravenous contrast is given in cases of suspected cerebral infarction.

73 In CT of the larynx:

A. Scans are made during suspended inspiration.
B. The piriform sinuses are filled out by the Valsalva manoeuvre.
C. 10 mm thick slices are usually obtained.
D. The canthomeatal line is at 90 degrees to the horizontal.
E. Asymmetry of the valleculae is abnormal.

Answers overleaf

72A
FALSE—Grey matter has a density of 35–40 units, and white matter a density about 10 less than this. Reference *B*, p. 341 (Fig. 24-21).

72B
TRUE—Reference *B*, p. 341 (Fig. 24-21).

72C
TRUE

72D
FALSE—It is about 1 rad, with a maximum of 1.6 rad. Reference *B*, p. 346.

72E
FALSE—It may result in a deterioration of the patient's condition.

73A
FALSE—They are made during a slow inspiratory effort. They are occasionally made during phonation ('e'). Reference *Q*, p. 37.

73B
TRUE—Reference *Q*, p. 40.

73C
FALSE—Contiguous slices 5 mm thick are obtained. Reference *Q*, p. 37.

73D
FALSE—The neck is extended 25–30 degrees to make the larynx as parallel to, and the vocal cords as perpendicular to, the table top as possible. Reference *Q*, p. 37.

73E
FALSE—This is a normal variant. Reference *Q*, p. 39.

74 In CT scans of the larynx:

A. The vocal processes of the arytenoid cartilages cannot be defined.
B. Soft-tissue density is normally recorded within the lumen of the cricoid ring.
C. The laryngeal ventricle can be usually seen separating the true and false cords.
D. The cricoid lamina has a medullary centre.
E. Fat usually fills the space anterior and lateral to the epiglottis.

75 In CT:

A. An intravenous or intraductal injection of contrast is required to demonstrate the parotid gland.
B. Iothalamate 320 is a suitable contrast agent for intraductal use in the parotid.
C. The infraorbital–meatal line is aligned parallel to the slice plane in scanning of the paranasal sinuses.
D. Dental amalgum creates artefacts that preclude the examination of facial structures.
E. The thyroid gland appears dense because of its contained iodine.

Answers overleaf

74A
FALSE—They are seen in 50% of patients. They define the level of the true cords. Reference *Q*, p. 42.

74B
FALSE—This would indicate tumour. Normally, no intraluminal soft-tissue density is appreciable at the level of the cricoid because the mucosa is adherent to the cartilage. Reference *Q*, p. 41.

74C
FALSE—The laryngeal ventricle is seen in this way in only 10% of scans. This is a weakness of CT and it may be difficult to ascertain the spread of tumour from false to true cords or vice versa. Reference *Q*, p. 49.

74D
TRUE—Situated within a dense cortical rim. Reference *Q*, p. 41.

74E
TRUE—The fat in the so-called pre-epiglottic and paralaryngeal spaces is well demonstrated by CT. The spaces become obliterated by deeply infiltrating neoplasm which has a much higher density. Reference *Q*, p. 43.

75A
FALSE—The parotid has a relatively low density because of contained fat. Masses associated with it are usually seen on an unenhanced scan. Contrast enhancement is sometimes helpful. Reference *N*, 22.1, p. 147.

75B
FALSE—It is too dense and liable to produce artefacts. A medium with a low iodine concentration (5–7%) is required. Reference *N*, 22.1, p. 147.

75C
TRUE—Additional scans may be performed in the coronal plane. Reference *N*, 22.1, p. 107.

75D
FALSE—However, it will require that the plane of cut be changed. Reference *N*, 22.1, p. 111.

75E
TRUE—It also enhances strongly after administration of intravenous contrast. Reference *Q*, p. 74.

76 In CT of the thorax:

A. Air is rarely demonstrated in the oesophagus.
B. Scans are made during suspended inspiration.
C. Short scanning times are important.
D. The oblique fissures are not visible.
E. Filling defects in the superior vena cava are seen in the normal patient during contrast enhancement.

77 In paediatric radiology:

A. Cold barium should be used for filling the oesophagus in suspected tracheo-oesophageal fistula.
B. Enema reduction of an intussusception may be performed in the presence of plain film evidence of small-bowel obstruction.
C. Enema reduction of an intussusception is performed with a hydrostatic pressure of 4–5 ft (1.22–1.53 m).
D. Leakage of contrast around the catheter should be avoided when filling the bladder at cystography.
E. The prone position is preferred for lumbar puncture in infants aged under 2 years.

Answers overleaf

76A
FALSE—Air is seen in the oesophagus in about 80% of normal patients. Reference *Q*, p. 59.

76B
TRUE—Variations in the phase of respiration may have a marked influence on CT appearances. Reference *Q*, p. 68.

76C
TRUE—In order to reduce artefacts from respiratory and cardiac motion. Reference *Q*, p. 68.

76D
FALSE—They may be seen. Reference *Q*, p. 66 (Fig. 16).

76E
TRUE—They result from the incomplete mixing of opacified and unopacified blood. They are more likely to be seen in the later scans of a dynamic series. Reference *Q*, p. 70.

77A
FALSE—Cardiac arrest may occur if the contrast is not warmed first to body temperature. Reference *S*, p. 325.

77B
FALSE—It is contra-indicated in this situation, and in the presence of shock or peritonitis. Reference *S*, p. 328.

77C
FALSE—The reduction should be attempted with the barium column no more than 1 m above the table. Reference *S*, p. 329.

77D
FALSE—This is a useful sign that adequate filling has occurred such that the child is likely to continue to micturate. Flexing of the toes is a similarly useful sign. Reference *S*, p. 334.

77E
TRUE—With the lumbar spine flexed over a pad. Reference *S*, p. 331.

78 In a perfusion lung scan:

A. The scintillation detectors consist of pure sodium iodide.
B. Scans are performed with particles 10–50 μm in size.
C. Counting is performed with the patient erect.
D. 40 000 counts are collected per image.
E. 1–3 mCi of activity is injected.

79 In scanning of the brain with radiopharmaceuticals:

A. No patient preparation is necessary when using sodium pertechnetate.
B. ^{99m}Tc-DTPA can be used.
C. Labelled glucoheptonate can be used.
D. The venous sinuses are not generally visible on a dynamic scan.
E. Delayed images should be obtained if a chronic subdural collection is suspected.

Answers overleaf

78A
FALSE—A controlled amount of thallium is added to the crystal. Reference *D*, p. 1.

78B
TRUE—^{99m}Tc-albumin macroaggregates or microspheres. Reference *D*, p. 17.

78C
FALSE—The patient should be supine because the pulmonary blood flow to the bases is increased in the erect position. Reference *D*, p. 85.

78D
FALSE—400 000 counts are collected. Reference *D*, p. 85.

78E
TRUE—Reference *D*, p. 85.

79A
FALSE—400 mg sodium or potassium perchlorate is given a half-hour before the injection to prevent uptake by the choroid plexuses and salivary glands. Reference *D*, p. 26.

79B
TRUE—The advantages being that no patient preparation is required and that there is a reduced radiation exposure (because of rapid renal elimination). Reference *D*, p. 25.

79C
TRUE—Reference *D*, p. 25.

79D
FALSE—The venous sinuses are seen after the arterial phase. The superior sagittal sinus is particularly prominent. Reference *D*, p. 28.

79E
TRUE—Late scans (at 4 hours) provide a diagnostic sensitivity of greater than 90% in the detection of chronic subdural haematoma. Reference *D*, p. 34.

80 In a technetium brain scan:

A. 2–3 mCi of pertechnetate is used.
B. Recent surgery or skin trauma may give false-positive results.
C. Cerebral secondaries are seen as areas of increased uptake on a dynamic scan.
D. Steroids reduce tracer uptake by neoplasms.
E. The ventricles are normally seen.

81 The following tracers are taken up by infarcted heart muscle:

A. [^{123}I]-hexadecanoic acid.
B. Potassium–43.
C. [^{99m}Tc]-glucoheptonate.
D. Thallium–201.
E. [^{99m}Tc]-pyrophosphate.

Answers overleaf

80A
FALSE—The dose is in the region of 15 mCi. Reference *D*, p. 27.

80B
TRUE—It is important to examine the patient in this situation. Reference *D*, p. 35.

80C
FALSE—They are usually silent at this stage. They produce areas of increased uptake on a static scan at a later stage. Reference *D*, p. 31.

80D
TRUE—So that it is desirable to perform the test before steroid therapy has been started. Reference *D*, p. 26.

80E
FALSE—Unless perchlorate has been omitted from the patient's preparation. Reference *D*, p. 26.

81A
FALSE—It concentrates in normal muscle so that infarcted muscle produces a 'cold spot'. Reference *D*, p. 59.

81B
FALSE—It produces a cold spot. Reference *D*, p. 59.

81C
TRUE—Forming a 'hot spot'. Reference *D*, p. 59.

81D
FALSE—It produces a cold spot. Reference *D*, p. 59.

81E
TRUE—It is widely used. Reference *D*, p. 60.

82 In scanning of the liver and spleen with radiopharmaceuticals:

A. Sulphur colloid is taken up by hepatocytes.
B. The spleen cannot be selectively imaged.
C. HIDA is seen in the gut at 20 minutes.
D. The gall bladder may normally be 'silent' in a HIDA scan in the fasting subject.
E. The total body radiation dose from a sulphur colloid scan is in the order of 1–2 rad (0.01–0.02 Gy).

83 In isotope renography:

A. [^{131}I]-hippuran is excreted largely by glomerular filtration.
B. DMSA is largely excreted by tubular secretion.
C. DTPA is excreted by glomerular filtration.
D. Sulphur colloid is used for blood-background subtraction.
E. The peak of the renogram curve is normally reached in 2–4 minutes.

Answers overleaf

82A
FALSE—It is taken up by the reticuloendothelial system (Reference *D*, p. 104). HIDA is taken up by hepatocytes.

82B
FALSE—Labelled, heat-damaged red blood cells can be used to image the spleen alone. Reference *D*, p. 117.

82C
TRUE—Reference *D*, p. 115.

82D
FALSE—A silent gall bladder is virtually diagnostic of acute cholecystitis. Reference *D*, p. 115.

82E
FALSE—It is 0.03–0.06 rad. Reference *Z*6, p. 97 (Table 7-7).

83A
FALSE—80% of the dose is eliminated by tubular secretion; the remainder is accounted for by filtration. Reference *D*, p. 137.

83B
TRUE—Reference *D*, p. 137.

83C
TRUE—Reference *D*, p. 137.

83D
FALSE—Human serum albumin, which is a blood-pool marker, is used. Reference *D*, p. 122.

83E
TRUE—A difference of greater than 1 minute between the kidneys in reaching the peak is considered to be indicative of unilateral disease. Reference *D*, p. 123.

84 In scintigraphy:

A. Anatomic markers are used in liver scans.
B. ^{99m}Tc-pyrophosphate is used to detect infarcted heart muscle within 6 hours of the infarction.
C. Cerebrospinal studies may be performed with ^{111}I-DTPA.
D. Markedly raised pulmonary end-diastolic pressures are a contra-indication to the performance of a perfusion scan.
E. The liver and spleen are seen on the normal bone scan.

85 ^{81m}Krypton:

A. Is used in cerebral blood flow studies.
B. Has a half-life of 5.5 days.
C. Emits radiation with energy of 191 keV.
D. Is taken up by the normal liver.
E. Is derived from thallium.

Answers overleaf

84A
TRUE—To mark the lower costal margin and the site of palpable abdominal masses. Markers are also important in thyroid scans. Reference *D*, p. 104.

84B
FALSE—This demonstrates infarcted muscle usually between 12 and 36 hours after the event. Thallium will show an infarct within the first 6 hours. Reference *D*, p. 60.

84C
TRUE—This is commonly used. Reference *D*, p. 38.

84D
FALSE—Perfusion scans are safe, although care should be taken in carrying out the study in the markedly compromised patient. Reference *D*, p. 84.

84E
FALSE—This may happen in the presence of reduced Tc-tin oxide impurity. Reference *D*, p. 21.

85A
TRUE—It is also used in lung ventilation scans. Reference *D*, p. 39.

85B
FALSE—It has a half-life of 13 seconds. Xenon–133 has a half-life of 5.5 days. Reference *D*, p. 39.

85C
TRUE—Reference *D*, p. 86.

85D
FALSE

85E
FALSE—It is obtained from rubidium–81. This has a short half-life (4.7 hours) which creates difficulties in obtaining a krypton generator. Reference *Z7*, p. 418.

86 The Valsalva manoeuvre:

A. Is used to demonstrate a swallowed foreign body lodged in the neck.
B. Is helpful when examining the oesophagus for varices.
C. Is used in myelography.
D. Improves the demonstration of superficial veins in lower limb venography.
E. Increases the subglottic angle in the larynx.

87 Lignocaine:

A. Is excreted unchanged by the kidneys.
B. Causes perioral paraesthesia and muscle tremor when an overdose is given.
C. Can cause convulsions.
D. Should not be given to patients on propranolol.
E. Interacts adversely with tricyclic antidepressants.

Answers overleaf

86A
TRUE—It is frequently difficult to separate ossification in the thyroid cartilage from that of an impacted fish bone. This problem is usually resolved by taking a lateral film of the neck before and during the Valsalva manoeuvre. The thyroid cartilage moves anteriorly, whilst a radio-opaque foreign body will be unchanged in position. Reference: Hadley, M.D.M. Letter to the editor. *British Medical Journal*; **289**:762 (1984).

86B
TRUE—Reference *S*, p. 15.

86C
FALSE

86D
FALSE—The manoeuvre helps to show the valves and improves the filling of deep veins such as the deep femoral and internal iliac veins. Incompetent communicating veins, particularly in the subsartorial canal, may be demonstrated during the performance of the manoeuvre. Reference *L*, p. 31.

86E
FALSE—It squares the angle. Reference *K*, p. 104.

87A
FALSE—It is broken down by the liver (Reference *V*, p. 380). In theory, adverse effects are more likely to occur with lignocaine when it is used in patients with severe liver disease.

87B
TRUE—Reference *Z*8, p. 781.

87C
TRUE—Reference *Z*8, p. 781.

87D
FALSE—No adverse interaction occurs.

87E
FALSE

88 A person who is taking monoamine oxidase inhibitors (MAOI):

A. Should not have arch aortography.
B. Should not receive intravenous glucose during angiography.
C. Should not be given adrenaline.
D. Can be given pethidine safely.
E. Should not be given barbiturates.

Answers overleaf

88A
FALSE—Angiography is not contra-indicated in patients taking MAOI.

88B
FALSE

88C
FALSE—Adrenaline can be given to patients on MAOI without its effects being potentiated. This is because it is chiefly destroyed by catechol-O-methyl transferase, and not by MAO. MAOI potentiate the indirect sympathomimetics, i.e. those that have their effect through the release of noradrenaline from nerve endings. Tyramine is the most noted example of such a drug. Reference *V*, p. 526.

88D
FALSE—Although pethidine is not metabolized by MAO, its effects on the central nervous system are potentiated by the inhibitors. Respiratory depression, restlessness and coma may result. Reference *V*, p. 528.

88E
TRUE—Because they potentiate the effects of barbiturates. Reference *V*, p. 528.

References

A. *Fundamental Physics of Radiology* by Meredith, W. J. and Massey, J. B. 3rd edition. John Wright and Sons, Bristol. 1977.

B. *Christensen's Introduction to the Physics of Diagnostic Radiology* by Curry, S. T., Dowdey, J. E. and Murry, R. C. 3rd edition. Lea and Febiger, Philadelphia. 1984.

C. *Radioisotopes in Radiodiagnosis* by Bligh, A. S., Leach, K. G. and Rhys Davies, E. 1st edition. Butterworths, London. 1976.

D. *Nuclear Medicine: An Introductory Text* by Ell, P. J. and Williams, E. S. 1st edition. Blackwell Scientific Publications, Oxford, 1981.

E. *A Textbook of Radiology and Imaging* edited by Sutton, D. 3rd edition. Churchill-Livingstone, Edinburgh. 1980.

F. *Practical Abdominal Ultrasound* by Metreweli, C. 1st edition. William Heinemann Medical Books, London. 1978.

G. *Essential Anatomy* by Lumley, J. S. P., Craven, J. L. and Aitken, J. T. 3rd edition. Churchill-Livingstone, Edinburgh. 1980.

H. *An Atlas of Anatomy Basic to Radiology* by Meschan, I. 1st edition. W. B. Saunders, Philadelphia. 1975.

I. *Double Contrast Gastrointestinal Radiology with Endoscopic Correlation* edited by Laufer, I. W. B. Saunders, Philadelphia. 1979.

J. *Practical Procedures in Diagnostic Radiology* by Saxton, H. M. and Strickland, B. 2nd edition. H. K. Lewis and Co., London. 1972.

K. *Interventional Diagnostic and Therapeutic Procedures* by Katzen, B. T. 1st edition. Springer-Verlag, New York. 1980.

L. *Phlebography of the Lower Limb* by Lea Thomas, M. 1st edition. Churchill-Livingstone, Edinburgh. 1982.

M. *Clinics in Obstetrics and Gynaecology: Ultrasound in Obstetrics and Gynaecology*, Vol. 10, No. 3., edited by Campbell, S. W. B. Saunders, Philadelphia. 1983.

N. *The Radiologic Clinics of North America*. W. B. Saunders, Philadelphia.

P1. *Cunningham's Manual of Practical Anatomy*, Vol. 1, 13th edition.

P2. *Cunningham's Manual of Practical Anatomy*, Vol. 2, 13th edition.

P3. *Cunningham's Manual of Practical Anatomy*, Vol. 3, 13th edition. Revised by Romanes, G. J. Oxford University Press. 1966.

Q. *Computed Body Tomography* by Lee, J. K. T., Sagel, S. S. and Stanley, R. J. 1st edition. Raven Press, New York. 1983.

R. *Clark's Positioning in Radiography*, edited by Kreel, L. Vol. 1, 10th edition. William Heinemann Medical Books, London. 1979.

S. *Techniques in Diagnostic Radiology* edited by Whitehouse, G. H. and Worthington, B. S. 1st edition. Blackwell Scientific Publications, Oxford. 1983.

T. *Basic Clinical Ultrasound* by Meire, H. and Farrant, P. British Institute of Radiology Teaching Series, No. 4. 1982.

U. *Complications in Diagnostic Radiology* edited by Ansell, G. 1st edition. Blackwell Scientific Publications, Oxford. 1976.

V. *Clinical Pharmacology* by Laurence, D. R. and Bennett, P. N. 5th edition. Churchill-Livingstone, Edinburgh. 1980.

W. *Chest Roentgenology* by Felson, B. 1st edition. W. B. Saunders, Philadelphia. 1973.

X. *Atlas of Normal Roentgen Variants That May Simulate Disease* by Keats, T. E. 3rd edition. Year Book Medical Publishers, New York. 1984.

Y. *Radiographic Photography and Imaging Processes* by Jenkins, D. 1st edition. MTP Press, Lancaster. 1980.

Z. *Code of Practice for the Protection of Persons Against Ionizing Radiations Arising from Medical and Dental Use.* HMSO, London. 1972.

Z1. *A Guide to Radiological Procedures* by Chapman, S. and Nakielny, R. Baillière Tindall, London. 1981.

Z2. *Nuclear Medicine—A Clinical Introduction* by Maisey, M. Update Books, London. 1980.

Z3. *Clark's Positioning in Radiography*, edited by Kreel, L. Vol. 2, 10th edition. William Heinemann Medical Books, London. 1979.

Z4. *Principles of Chest X-ray Diagnosis* by Simon, G. 3rd edition. Butterworths, London. 1971.

Z5. *Seminars in Roentgenology*. Pelvimetry Revisited, Vol. xvii, No. 3 by Bean, W. G. J. and Rodan, B. A. Grune and Stratton, Orlando, Florida. 1982.

Z6. *Introductory Physics of Nuclear Medicine* by Chandra, R. 2nd edition. Lea and Febiger, Philadelphia. 1982.

Z7. *Clinical Nuclear Medicine* by Maisey, M. N., Britton, K. E. and Gilday, D. L. Chapman and Hall, London. 1983.

Z8. *The Pharmacological Basis of Therapeutics* by Gilman, G. A., Goodman, L. S. and Gilman A. 6th edition. Macmillan, Basingstoke. 1980.